D0942691

THE A-Z OF
MEDICAL WRITING

MEDICAL LIBRARY
NATIONAL JEWISH
1400 Jackson St.
Denver, CO 80206

Tim Albert learnt the long words studying psychology and the short ones as a *Daily Mirror* trainee. He then worked for the broadsheets and the BBC and was education correspondent of the *New Statesman*. Rampant hypochondriasis steered him into medical journalism, and he was executive editor of *World Medicine* and editor of *BMA News Review*. Since 1990 he has run his own training company, delivering hundreds of courses on writing to doctors and other health professionals. He is a fellow of the Institute of Personnel and Development, organiser of the *BMJ*'s annual short course for journal editors, and visiting fellow in medical writing at Southampton University.

THE A-Z OF MEDICAL WRITING

Tim Albert
Tim Albert Training, Surrey, UK

BMJ
Books

© BMJ Books 2000
BMJ Books is an imprint of the BMJ Publishing Group

All rights reserved. No part of this book may be reproduced, stored in a retrieval system or transmitted, in any form or by any means, electronic, mechanical, photocopying, recording and/or otherwise, without the prior permission of the publishers.

First published in 2000
Reprinted 2001
by BMJ Books, BMA House, Tavistock Square,
London WC1H 9JR

www.bmjbooks.com

British Library Cataloguing in Publication Data

A catalogue record for this book is available from the British Library

ISBN: 0-7279-1487-1

Typeset by Saxon Graphics, Derby
Printed and bound in Great Britain by J. W. Arrowsmith Ltd, Bristol

Contents

Foreword

This book has not been written to be read – at least in the usual sense of starting at the beginning, ploughing on to the end, and then remembering (at best) one or two points. I have written it for a completely different purpose, which has come from my experiences over the past 10 years working with doctors and other health professionals to sort out a wide range of writing problems.

It is clear that they face several difficulties when it comes to writing. They are torn between the pressure to communicate with patients on the one hand, and meet the expectations of their peers for horrendously prolix prose on the other. Although they will have had no formal training on writing since they were 16, they will be expected to publish in high status journals if they are to advance in their careers. Writing cultures have grown up that are, frankly, destructive of effective communication and individual talent. And of course, as trained doctors rather than trained writers, they have more useful things to do anyway.

So this is not another reference book laying down rules on grammar, style, or journalology, or the presentation of statistics or the ethics of publication, even though I stray into these areas from time to time. What this book sets out to do is to give support, encouragement, and informed advice, so that people who have found writing hard will somehow find it less hard. Acting on the experience of training courses, I have chosen a large number of topics, which are arranged alphabetically, from **abbreviations** to **zzzzz**.

Tim Albert

FOREWORD

How to use this book

I expect this book to be used in two ways. The first is as an old-fashioned companion, to be kept by a bedside or on a desk, so that you can dip into it during an otherwise idle moment and find the odd entry that will interest, amuse, stimulate or annoy. The second is to use it for advice and encouragement when you have a specific writing problem. You have been asked to write an obituary, for instance, or you are suffering from writer's block. In such cases, you should turn to the specific entry, which in turn should guide you to other related entries, and in some cases to details of books that I have on my bookshelf and find useful. A word in **bold type** shows that there is another section also of use.

This book, as the title makes clear, is a personal choice, and I am sure that many topics could have been dealt with differently, and that some important ones have been left out altogether. I hope that this book will evolve, and that we shall be able to make regular updates, both in the paper version and in electronic form. To that end I hope that readers will send me their comments, including suggestions for new items to be covered in the next edition, and other pieces of advice and comment.

Finally I would like to thank all those who have helped, in their various ways, with this book. These are Gordon Macpherson, Harvey Marcovitch, Pete Moore, Geoff Watts, Geert-Jan van Daal, Don Rowntree, Margaret Hallendorff, Mary Banks and Michèle Clarke. The person who has suffered most for my art, as always, has been my wife Barbara, to whom I offer my special thanks.

Tim Albert
Dorking
tatraining@compuserve.com

A–Z of Medical Writing

Abbreviations   Modern science writing is written increasingly in a kind of code, littered with phrases such as 'a breakthrough in PE' and 'no laboratory monitoring of APT'. Proponents argue that this is inevitable; it reflects the increasing specialization of medicine and saves valuable space for yet more papers.

Opponents say that abbreviations mislead and confuse. One person's British Medical Association will be another's British Midland Airways, or (as I once saw in a conference hotel in America) a Branch Marketing Assistant. The initials CIA are identified so closely with US spies that it may be difficult to remember that they also stand for common iliac arteries. The confusion intensifies when the abbreviations disappear for a while, only to resurface after an absence of several paragraphs when you have completely forgotten what they stand for. For this reason, and because they are in upper case, they slow the reader down. They also send a strong message to the reader: this is our language, if you are uncomfortable with it, you don't belong.

Those who want to avoid abbreviations can usually do so, for instance by spelling out in full one of the component words: 'the association', 'the airline' or 'the assistant'. If you do insist on using abbreviations, make sure that you spell out the words in full at their first appearance, and try to use no more than two sets per document (*see* **acronyms; political writing**).

Absolutes   Many people use phrases such as 'absolute perfection' and 'completely exhausted', where the first word is redundant (though not 'totally redundant'!). *See also* **tautology.**

Abstracts   There are two types of abstracts. There are those that stand on their own, as a means of securing an invitation to present at a conference. I call these **conference abstracts** and they have an entry to themselves (*see below*).

The other type are those that appear at the start of a scientific paper, summarizing the information contained in that paper. According to the **Vancouver Group**, an abstract should state the purposes of the study or investigation, basic procedures, main findings, and the principal conclusions: 'It should emphasize new and important aspects of the study or observation'. In some respects they are a marketing tool,

1

enabling potential readers to decide whether they should read the paper in detail. With the development of electronic databases, they now have a role as a stand-alone unit of scientific knowledge.

Approach writing an abstract in the same way as you would approach any other writing task (*see* **process of writing**). Don't just try to cut your article back to fit the space available, but treat this as a separate piece of writing. There are two pitfalls to avoid.

- *Ignoring the specifications.* Journals will make it absolutely clear in the **Instructions to Authors** how they like their abstract to appear, and it is senseless to ignore these requirements. A modern trend is the structured abstract, which has carefully defined sections to complete. Study the instructions carefully, and look at abstracts in your target journal. One of the most commonly flouted requirements is length: if they say 300 words they mean 300 words; any more may be cut and your work could become meaningless.

- *Deviating from the original.* It is not hard to find examples of submitted (and sometimes published) articles where details in the abstract simply do not appear in the article itself. This danger is particularly acute when the abstract has been written first. By the time the paper has been written and the co-authors have agreed, all kind of subtle changes have been made.

Acceptance   The supreme moment when something you have written is accepted for publication. Treasure it.

Acknowledgements   According to the **Vancouver Group** these are the statements accompanying a scientific paper that 'specify (a) contributions that do not justify authorship, such as general support by a department chair, (b) acknowledgements of technical help, (c) acknowledgements of financial and material support, which should specify the nature of the support; and (d) relationships that may pose a conflict of interest'. Naming people in this way assumes that they endorse the contents, so you must have their written permission. Technical help should be acknowledged in a separate paragraph. Journals will vary in their approach to this (*see* **Instructions to Authors**). The word can have a slightly different meaning when it comes to books. In such instances it is used to acknowledge **Copyright** material.

Acronyms   These are **abbreviations** that can be pronounced as a word, and are currently the fashionable way to describe (and market) a piece of science – the ARIC study, the HOT trial or just plain MONICA. The number is exploding, so if you want to use one, make sure it has not already been taken.

Many newspapers and magazines adopt the style that, if you can pronounce an acronym, you write it with one initial capital only. Thus UN but Unesco. This explains why, although AIDS seems to be the preferred style in medical journals, most other publications style it Aids. Both are right, within their contexts (*see* **style guides**).

Action lists   These are beginning to take over from the more traditional **minutes** as the preferred way of recording the activities of a committee. They are based on the principle that recording the decisions is fairly straightforward; the hard thing is ensuring that they are carried out. To produce an action list, write down in clear **active** language, what has to be done, by whom, and by when. Review at the start of each meeting.

Active   The basic way of writing a sentence, in which someone or something does something to someone or something else. Thus: 'Dr Smith wrote the article' and 'The article changed the world'. The place of the active in science writing is confused and controversial (*see* **verbs; voice**).

Adjectives   Describing words, such as 'old', 'busy'. We overuse them dreadfully: 'When you catch an adjective, kill it', said Mark Twain. Say exactly how old ('41 years and a day'), or how we can tell that the person was busy ('Between lunch and tea she chaired three meetings, ran four miles on the treadmill, and attended a bar mitzvah').

Adverbs   The words that modify a verb (or 'doing' word), such as 'slowly', 'quickly'. Again, these can be overused. Prefer **nouns** and **verbs**: 'He took four hours to answer the question.'

Advertising   Written material that promotes the interests of whoever paid for it. Distinguish from **editorial**.

3

Advertorial   Articles that look like objective text, but are in fact paid for by an advertiser. They appear more frequently in smaller, local publications, and can usually be recognized by the large number of favourable **adjectives**: 'elegant surroundings', 'friendly staff', 'mouthwatering desserts'. Editors should make it clear that these are advertising features but, alas, do not always do so.

Advice on writing   You will have little difficulty finding people to comment on what you have written. The problem is knowing when their advice is useful – or ill-informed and dangerous. Beware those who base their comments on their own views on 'good writing' without finding out how you have defined your **audience** and what you want your writing to achieve (*see* **false feedback loop**). Good advisers will first ask for details of your target audience. They will also give you **balanced feedback**.

Agents   One of the most common questions that would-be writers ask is: 'Should I get an agent?'. The best answer is to turn it round: 'Should an agent spend time on you?'. What do you offer that will give enough income for two to share?

If you believe that you are about to make huge amounts of money from your writing and want some help in getting the best deal, there are two main ways of finding an agent. The first is to get a reference book (*see below*), look up the names of some agents, and identify one or two that sound suitable. This process is unlikely to be scientific. You will then have to send in some kind of proposal. Your chances of being accepted by the first agent, or even any agent, are slight. An alternative technique is to find and bedazzle one at a party: this means joining the kind of group where these people are likely to congregate, such as the Society of Authors.

Meanwhile, don't give up the day job.

BOOKLIST: agents
- *Writers' and artists' yearbook*, London: A&C Black, 1999. First published in the first decade of the 20th century, this has nearly 700 pages packed with names, addresses and other information, plus useful articles on a range of topics from copyright to research and the Internet.

- *The writer's handbook*, edited by Barry Turner, London: Macmillan 1999. A more recent guide, with 750 pages packed with similar information. All this and a foreword from PD James.

American English
This can give problems (*see* **UK–US English**).

Amongst
A curiously old-fashioned word. What's wrong with 'among'?

Analytical skills
These are at the heart of good writing. Unless you have a clear idea of the **message** you wish to put across, you are merely collecting data and shuffling it around (*see* **leaf shuffling; process of writing**).

And
You are allowed to start a sentence with this word (and with 'But'). And those who tell you otherwise are ill-informed. But if they don't believe you, invite them to look in any contemporary reference work (*see* **grammar booklist**).

Annual report of public health
Public health departments have to publish an annual report. Unfortunately nobody really made it clear why and – more importantly – for whom. While the best reports give clear, considered messages to specified audiences – such as professional colleagues, local politicians, or the *Guardian*-reading public – many fall uncomfortably between a number of audiences, pleasing none and costing a fair amount of money and aggravation.

This confusion has a clear implication. Directors of public health must clearly assume, or assign to another, the role of **editor** for their annual report. This means defining and communicating the report's **mission** and primary audience, which will enable their colleagues to write their chapters effectively, using last year's report as a model (*see* **evidence-based writing**). This in turn should free everybody to get on with some of the better defined tasks in public health.

Antipathy   The feeling that readers have for pieces of writing that are over-long, over-researched, and over-written (*see* **PIANO**).

Apathy   A frequent cry among editors is: 'No one will bother writing for me!'. Why should they (*see* **commissioning**)?

Apostrophes   Rarely does the wrong use of the apostrophe change the meaning of a sentence. But it is an error that some people seize upon with glee, inferring that whoever made it must be ill-educated, incompetent and therefore can be ignored. Writers should make every effort to get it right; it's not particularly difficult because its solution is at hand.

When it comes to the difference between 'its' and 'it's', forget about learning about possessives and so on (if you don't know now you probably never will). Simply consider the apostrophe as the top of an 'i'. Thus 'it's colour' really means 'it is colour' ('It is colour that makes the difference' as opposed to 'Its colour is red'). This should help you to get it right. If you still don't understand, ask people who know about these things to check them for you (*see* **grammar booklist**).

Appendix   Additional material that comes at the end of a report, but is an optional extra: a useful device because it offers readers the opportunity to see the evidence without having to plough through it all.

Article   A piece of writing that is published. There are two types: those published in magazines and newspapers (*see* **feature article**), or those published in journals (*see* **scientific paper**). Confuse the two at your peril. *See also* **review articles; short articles**.

Audience   The person or persons for whom you are writing. The chances of your work being read increase dramatically if you follow the following two principles.
- *Define the audience tightly.* When writing a letter, you can target the recipient. When writing a report, you can target the decision maker. When writing for a publication, you can target the editor.

- *Separate distinct audiences.* It becomes much harder to make a piece of writing work when you have to balance the needs of distinct audiences, such as a panel of doctors and a group of patients. If you have two audiences, do two pieces of writing. The time needed to write the second version will be far less than you fear, but the chances of getting the message across will increase significantly.

This is probably one of the great principles of effective writing. If you have a clear idea of your readers, you can research what style and structure works for them (*see* **evidence based writing**).

Author's editors   A few academic departments throughout the world employ professional **technical editors** to help doctors and scientists to prepare a paper for publication. Although there are some excellent practitioners, the system has failed to take off.

One of the main reasons is that employing someone who knows about writing is helpful only if those who employ them are equally as informed. Often good advice from the author's editor is over-ruled, wasting time and money. And if a paper is turned down, it's the author's editor, not the author, who tends to get the blame.

Authorship   Over the past few years the question of authorship – whether someone has his or her name attached as a 'part owner' of a scientific paper – has become a hot issue. This is because the way editors tend to define it is at odds with the way it is defined by the authors themselves.

Editors are vehemently opposed to the practice of listing people as co-authors when they have contributed little or nothing (**gift authorship**). The **Vancouver Group** clearly states that each author 'should have participated sufficiently in the work to take public responsibility for the content. Authorship credit should be based only on substantial contributions ... Participation solely in the acquisition of funding or the collection of data does not justify authorship.'

Things look different from the author's point of view, and these principles are of little help to junior doctors, who are not in a position to argue when seniors demand to be included on the list of authors. Usually they have no choice but to add the name, even though the new 'author' contributed little or nothing. One useful technique is to agree on the number and role of the co-authors before

7

the article is written (*see* **brief setting**). This should limit the practice of people jumping aboard once all the work has been done.

The real cause of the trouble is the fact that authorship is now one of the main international performance indicators for scientists and, less obviously, for doctors. There is no reason to believe that the ability to publish in an English language journal should predict the clinical performance of a Dutch doctor, but that is currently a fact of life, and until the system is reformed conflicts will exist between those who want some easy points (and perhaps get back to their proper jobs) and editors who feel that this is somehow not playing the game.

Meanwhile, the current trend is for journals to add lists explaining who did what. If this is the style of your target journal, then follow it (*see* **evidence-based writing**). *See also* **ghost author**.

Autobiography   Great to do; don't expect others to be interested (*see* **vanity publishing**).

Bad writing   I take a pragmatic view and define bad writing as writing that fails to get the desired message across to the target audience (*see* **brief setting**). Four types of errors may get in the way.
- *It's wrong.* The writing may read easily and appear plausible but, alas, the arguments depend on facts that appear to be, or later turn out to be, not true (*see* **scientific fraud**). There is absolutely no defence for this.
- *The language is inappropriate.* The author has chosen words and constructions with which the audience is not familiar (*see* **jargon**). This can be fixed relatively easily, if the will is there.
- *It is difficult to follow the argument.* The sentences don't seem to follow on from one another, so that readers find it difficult to understand what is going on (*see* **structure; yellow marker test**). This can be fixed by altering sentences and paragraphs, though it takes considerable time and is difficult to do well.
- *It leaves the reader wondering why it was written at all.* These are those pieces of writing that you gamely wade through, but by the

end have no idea why (*see* **brief setting; message**). If the writer cannot define a clear message, then the reader will be unable to, and the writing will be doomed to fail.

Balanced feedback   When people ask us to comment on their writing, we tend to shower them with criticism (*see* **correcting the work of others**). Balanced feedback is a simple technique that allows us to improve the writing without wrecking the writer's morale.

Whenever you are asked your opinion on a piece of writing, first establish the **audience** for which is intended. Read the piece quickly, after which you will be in a position to make up your mind on the following key questions.

- *What is the message and is it right for the target audience?* Is the message in an appropriate place (look in particular at the first and last sentences). Is it a reasonable message? And is it appropriate for the audience?
- *Is the writing structured in an appropriate way?* Did the writing keep your interest or did you find yourself flagging? Were there places where you had to go back and start again?
- *Is the tone appropriate?* Ask whether the style is, broadly speaking, appropriate, but don't worry too much at this stage about individual points of **style**. Here the various **readability tests** will come in useful.

These are **macro-editing** issues, and you should be able to find at least one area where the writer has done well. Write a short note, drawing attention to what you think is already good – and what you think the writer needs to work on. For example: 'You have a clear message, which is interesting and well worth putting across to your target readers. You have written it in an appropriate tone. The argument became a little difficult to follow between the fifth and eighth paragraphs – and you may wish to insert some key sentences so that the reader can see why you have included this information.'

If you still wish to deface the text with detailed changes (**micro-editing**) you can now do so. You will have put them in context as fairly minor amendments (or nit-picking stuff). Even under these circumstances I would urge restraint: would it *really* make a difference if you didn't have your way over style every time? (*see* **macro-editing; micro-editing**).

Biorhythms   If you need to do a lot of writing, work out the best times of the day for you in which to write. If possible, arrange your schedule so that you can write during these periods: your writing is unlikely to be fresh and attractive if you are fighting an overwhelming desire to take a nap.

Block   *See* **writer's block.**

Blurb   A piece of writing that puffs itself or praises another, as on the outside of this book cover (I hope). Science journals increasingly carry blurbs (or short summaries of interesting articles) on an early editorial page. The purpose of these is to whip up interest and entice readers to keep turning the pages.

Booklists   A kind of fashion accessory, without which it appears no self-respecting book should be published. I suspect that few people make much use of them. This book does not have a booklist at the back. Instead I have chosen one or two books from my bookshelf and will recommend them at the appropriate point. Under **grammar,** for instance, there will be a short selection of books, for reading and reference.

Books, buying of   To be encouraged, though sadly the knowledge in them is not transferred unless they are actually read.

Book reviews   Follow the same principles as for **review articles,** but keep them shorter.

Books, editing of   In a fast-changing world, where one person will find it difficult to keep in touch with all the developments in even a narrow specialty, there is a good case for **multi-authored** books. But someone has to edit them. Those chosen may not have to spend hours researching topics just below the horizons of their immediate knowledge, but they will have a host of other problems. Here are some tips.

- *Be absolutely clear that you want to do the book.* Editing takes up huge amounts of time, and will eat into the rest of your life. It is flattering to be asked to edit a book, but what's in it for you? And what can you give up to make the time?
- *Establish good relations with the publishers.* Before you invest your time, make sure that you have a clear proposal from the publisher, and that you are happy with it. You may wish to take advice from a lawyer or (if you are a member) from a group such as the Society of Authors. Issues to clarify include the nature of rewards for you and your contributors, the amount of practical support (e.g. letters to contributors) that the publishers will provide, and (particularly important these days) electronic rights. Do not over-negotiate. Establishing a good relationship with the commissioning editor at this stage will pay off later. Consider lunch.
- *Make explicit plans.* Work out what topics you will need to cover, and decide who you want to cover them. Don't rely on your own network: literature searches will enable you to locate acknowledged experts. Work out a timetable, allowing plenty of slack for slow writers. Have a fallback plan – for instance another author standing by – for the inevitable authors who fail to deliver.
- *Brief the contributors.* Make sure everyone knows exactly what you want them to do, in what form and by when. Write down clearly what you want them to achieve (*see* **brief setting**). Make sure they know what the other contributors are covering and who the audience will be. Give clear **deadlines**. Make sure everything is in writing (*see* **commissioning**).
- *Support the contributors.* Many editors feel that once they have briefed their contributors, all they need to do is to pen an elegant introduction. This is an illusion. You should build in some support for your writers, such as a telephone call, otherwise the chances are you will reach the final deadline with no copy submitted (*see* **apathy**).
- *Collect the chapters and do some macro-editing.* Publishers will want their own technical editors to have an input, but there is still an important role for the editor in reading the submissions, making sure that they meet the intended purpose and standard, and sorting them out so that they do. Keep an eye out for unfair criticism of the work of rivals (*see* **defamation**); you may need to dig deep into your reserves of tact and diplomacy.
- *Thank the contributors.* Most will have spent time and effort on your behalf, so it is common courtesy to thank them as soon as they send in their chapter, with a follow-up letter and a copy of the

book once it is published. Apart from anything else, if you decide to do another book, you will need some good and loyal writers.

At the end many editors feel that they have written it all themselves. Sometimes they have.

Books, writing of

There are many good reasons why you should under no circumstances write a book. It eats time (as a rough guide equivalent to three months of a full-time job). It is difficult to find a publisher. It is a painful activity, during which writers become deeply antisocial. The financial rewards are usually low, and out of proportion to the work involved.

If, after reading this, you still want to continue, then you probably should. The first thing to do is to have an idea. Then ask the key question: will enough people be interested enough to spend money on buying it? If you still wish to keep going, follow these stages.

- *Identify a suitable publisher.* Go to a bookshop or use the Internet to browse, then construct a proposal, and send it in. Publishers are interested in good ideas, and want evidence that you are likely to do it well. Start with a brief description (200 words or so) of what you intend to do and who will buy the book. Include a list of chapter headings (for non-fiction) or a sample chapter (if fiction). You will also need a **covering letter,** giving perhaps one or two reasons why you think you should be trusted (author of 17 other books, professor of book writing, UN expert on pagination, etc). Finally, add supporting information, such as articles you may have written, or a **CV.** Send everything off, keeping a copy in the drawer. Now try to obliterate any trace of it from your memory until you receive the reply.
- *Gain from the pain.* Most people fail at the first attempt, so learn from **rejection.** Even if you think the publisher has made a dreadful mistake (and it does happen: George Orwell's manuscript for *Animal farm* was rejected on the grounds that it is 'impossible to sell animal stories in the USA'), consider whether you could and should make changes.
- *Accept your first contract graciously.* Your contract will almost certainly offer substantially less than you think you are worth. You may wish to consult a lawyer or the Society of Authors; alternatively you may wish to take the view that publishers are doing this all the time, and as a newcomer and first-time author it will be unwise to rock the boat. (After the extraordinary success of your first book, however, you can afford to take a more muscular line,

employ an **agent** and screw the publishers into the ground, if that is your style.

- *Sit down and plan.* Work out when you have to submit the manuscript and put the key dates in your diary. Work back: allow time for rewriting. Also allow time for other people to look at the manuscript, and for doing the tricky administrative things like seeking **copyright**. Then put down some **deadlines** for the actual writing: how many of your 50 000 words do you intend to write a month? And, more importantly, when? How will you find time – do you plan to give up your evenings at the gym, or your mornings in bed, or your weekends in the garden? (*see* **time management**).

- *Keep in touch with your editor.* It helps if your editor still has positive feelings towards you when you send in your manuscript. Don't be afraid to ask for advice: it is better to sort out problems early rather than haggle over them at the last minute.

- *Find out how your publisher would like the copy to be presented.* Most publishers like a 'clean' disk (i.e. simple text without designed tables and boxes; italics and bold are normally translated easily into other systems), so that their own **copy-editors** or designers can do the formatting (or 'marking up') themselves. But this does not necessarily mean that you have to write it that way. If, like me, you are one of those people who need to fiddle with the way your writing actually looks (see **layout**), feel free to do so.

- *When you finally send the manuscript off, expect changes.* Your publisher will have been involved in many more books than you have and will be better attuned to the target audience. This doesn't mean to say that copy editors are infallible, but if you do disagree, do so with tact, charm and, above all, evidence and a reasoned argument (evidence-based complaining?). If you think every proposed change is an insult to your great talent, you are either being unrealistic or are with the wrong publisher. You then have a simple decision to take: do you negotiate, or do you end the relationship and try to find another publisher?

- *Enjoy the publication.* After about six months the book will be published – and there will probably be an anticlimax. Do all you can to help during the marketing phase.

Now is the time to await the plaudits and the cheques. Both will offer meagre fare. Your friends will say (to your face) that the book is wonderful (and then drop hints about a free signed copy); letters of praise from unknown admirers are less likely. As for the money, you will probably have signed a contract for 12.5% net of the royalties. With a print run of, say, 2000 at a price of £12.50, that will give you about £1500 (less tax) if all copies are sold. Hardly a good return on the huge effort you made.

The real point about writing books is that, like mountains, they are there. Some of us cannot resist the challenge; but it's hardly rational behaviour.

Books, writing of chapters in   One of the great advantages of multi-authored books is that they meet the huge demand for authorship. But even single chapters require a major investment of time – a week's work or more to do it properly. Be flattered by the invitation to contribute, and then consider whether you really want (or need) to invest the time. Saying no at this stage will be appreciated: publishers say that their biggest problem in multi-authored books is dealing with the delays caused by those who keep insisting that they want to contribute, but never get around to doing so.

Approach the project as you would any other writing task (*see* **process of writing**). Divide the chapter into manageable chunks of 1000 words or so, and use the structure of a **feature article** for each section.

Your main reward will be satisfaction of a job well done. You are unlikely to get paid, and if so it will rarely be above £200 a chapter. You should be offered a free copy of the book; make sure you display it prominently.

Boredom   We often experience this when reading what others have written. Curiously, we never expect our readers to do so when reading our work.

Borrowing other people's ideas   This is stealing. Do not do it (*see* **copyright**; **plagiarism**).

Bosses   Some are marvellously helpful when it comes to giving **balanced feedback** on what we write. Others are discouraging, and sometimes dangerous. Remember that bosses can turn into a powerful **false feedback loop**, and that throughout the writing process our duty is to argue – tactfully – for the interests of our target readers (*see* **negotiating over copy**).

Brainstorming   Throughout the writing process our tendency to criticize can overwhelm our capacity to be creative. Brainstorming techniques try to circumvent that in the planning stage by encouraging us to put down our thoughts on paper – as they come and without stopping to criticize them. At its basic level we can use this method to compile a list. A development of this is **branching** (*see below*) where we allow our thoughts to spill out all over the page in a much freer way. A sophisticated version of this is **mindmapping**, a system developed by Tony Buzan (*see* **process of writing booklist**).

Branching   Branching techniques, such as spidercharts and **mindmapping**, play an important part in the writing process – in particular, at the stage when you have decided on your **message** and need to collect and arrange the information needed to prove it.

All you need is the message, a large piece of paper with at least one pen or pencil (some say more) and 5–10 minutes. Write the message in the middle of the paper ('All writers should buy a treadmill') and then start asking questions ('What kind of writers?', 'What kind of treadmill?', 'How should writers use it?' 'How do we know it helps?' and so on). Each question should lead to others, and when you come to the end of one train of thought you should go back to the message in the middle and start again. Within minutes you will have a page covered with words, all coming out from the message in the middle.

The advantage of this, as one course participant once put it, is that the mess in your head is now the mess on a piece of paper. This is a breakthrough. Committing yourself to putting things down on paper is one of the hardest parts of writing (*see* **writer's block**), but as soon as you have something down you can start to control it. You will, for instance, be able to distinguish between matters of substance that must be included, and detail that *could* be included if space permits. All will be related to the message.

Breaks   Locking yourself in a room for three hours at a time is unlikely to boost your creativity. Try to write in short bursts of, say, 10–15 minutes, and make sure that you really are writing and not worrying about what you have just written (*see* **free writing**).

15

Nothing benefits a piece of writing more than the temporary leaving of it. *See also* **time management.**

Brief setting   One of the great mistakes we make when writing is to start too early, without really knowing where we want to end up. Some people start by writing lists; others go straight to a word processor and start writing down what comes into their heads. I recommend an alternative step, originally recommended in *Medical journalism; the writer's guide* (*see* **Journalism booklist**), in which I advise that the first thing to do is to draw back from writing – and to think very carefully about what you want to do. By all means let your writing be a voyage of discovery, but look at the existing navigation charts before you set out.

I call this stage 'setting the brief'. It involves taking time to think about what you want to do. You may be able to do it in less than a minute; with more difficult pieces of writing you may need days or even weeks. As long as it remains **rumination**, not procrastination, you should not worry. As for what you need to think about, these are contained in the following five points.

- *Message.* Work out the most important thing you want your readers to take away from your writing. This is the **message,** and should take the form of a simple sentence of about 10 words. For instance: 'Wearing sandals with socks reduces the incidence of athlete's foot.' The key is to include a verb ('reduces', 'increases', 'does not affect', etc.) which gives it direction. It will also distinguish it from a **title,** which (in journals) usually consists of a string of nouns ('Footwear apparel and fungal infections of the skin and nails of the feet: a randomized placebo-controlled trial') that will not make a suitable starting point. Do not settle for a question: if you do not yet have the answer, do more research or more thinking or both.

- *Market.* Decide for whom this message is intended (**audience**) and how you intend to get it to them. Be specific: the more tightly defined your audience, the greater your chances of success. If you want to write an article, define which journal (*The Lancet*, for instance, or *Country Life*?). If you are writing a report justifying the purchase of an expensive piece of equipment, write for the main player in the decision-making committee. If you are writing a procedure for a new clinic's appointment system, write for those who will have to carry it out. If it looks as though you will have to please two separate audiences at the same time – such as a report on the latest research for members of a patient group and interested doctors – then write two different reports.

- *Length and other aspects of style.* Now work out what you need to please your audience. Decide on the length of the piece of writing, measured in words or **paragraphs**. This should not be determined by how you rate the importance of the topic (or happen to know about it), but on what the market should bear.
- *Deadlines.* Set the date by which you need to finish the writing. Then work backwards, inserting second-level **deadlines** for the major steps you need to take on the way.
- *Payoff.* Define how you will judge the success of your writing. Too often we judge it in terms of half-remembered notions of literary criticism (*see* **English teachers; examinations**). Now we are established in our careers, we should regard writing as a tool not a test, and therefore judge success not by the details, but by whether our writing has enabled us to achieve what we set out to do. For instance, if we are trying to attract a £1 million grant, and we manage to do so, our writing has succeeded, irrespective of whether we have split the odd infinitive. Similarly, if we are trying to get a paper published in a prestigious journal and it is accepted, we have also succeeded (and subsequent gripes from rivals should be seen in this context).

Take your time over brief setting. You may not believe it at the time, but having a clear idea on the above five questions will make all the difference to what you are setting out to do. Consider the following examples, both on the subject of socks, shoes and athlete's foot:

- *Task 1.* 'A research letter for *The Lancet* showing that sandals and socks reduce the incidence of athlete's foot. This will be based on the multicentre SOLE trial and will comprise 500 words. The article will be written by August 1, revised by August 15, sent out to co-authors on September 1 and submitted on September 21. The writing will be considered successful when the editor accepts it for publication.'
- *Task 2.* 'A report for the management board arguing that sandals and socks should be issued to all staff in order to reduce the incidence of athlete's foot. The primary audience will be the director of human resources. The report will consist of one sheet of A4. The first draft will be completed tomorrow, and revised the following day. The writing will be considered successful when staff get issued with their regulation socks and sandals.'

A useful trick is to make sure that others, such as **bosses** or **co-authors**, who may subsequently want to comment on your piece of writing, see these details before you start. Don't wait for the finished piece; show them the brief. Agreeing on the message and the market at this early stage can save endless arguments later on (*see* **negotiating over copy**).

Bullet points

Bullet points are currently fashionable. They are useful when:

- you have a small number of discrete facts, all of which are roughly as important as the others, and
- you expect your reader to be skimming what you have written.

They become less useful when you want to persuade or lead your readers through a complicated argument, or perhaps feel that your reader could do with a little entertainment.

There is a trap when it comes to punctuating bullet point lists. Strictly speaking the bullet is not a punctuation mark, so you should ignore it. A list should therefore start with a colon like this:

- not followed by a capital letter and not ending in a full stop but in a comma or semicolon,
- until you get to the last point.

Byline

The name of an author on an article in a newspaper or magazine. Getting one of these can be a major incentive (*see* **commissioning**).

Capital letters

These should be used for signalling the beginning of a sentence, or of a proper noun such as Aylesbury or Zimmerman. They need no longer be used for seasons, though they are still used for months and days of the week. Do *not* use them on the grounds that they make the word look more important (*see* **pompous initial capitals**).

Careers in writing   A number of jobs combine a knowledge of medical matters with an interest in writing. These include working as an associate editor on a scientific **journal**, working as a writer on a **medical newspaper** or producing marketing material for pharmaceutical companies. It is tempting to look at these as an escape route from the demands of patients and colleagues, and indeed working as a writer has a number of good points. Writing professionals tend to be less hierarchical, and the hours tend to be more civilized. You can see what you produce, and can measure your performance (*see* **effective writing**).

But being a doctor will not in itself qualify you to write about medicine, and you will need to acquire some extra skills. This could mean a full-time course for a year, or it could mean a period of apprenticeship within medical writing. The levels of pay are likely to be less than one would expect as a doctor. For further information contact doctors who are already working in these fields.

Case notes   Doctors are writing these all the time, yet they are difficult to do – and are often done badly. Tell the story, so that one week later (the next doctor) or five years later (the lawyers) will be able to reconstruct exactly what happened. Tell the truth, and write clearly.

Case reports   In the past these were a good way to get your name on the databases. Unfortunately the current trend for larger and larger statistical samples means that they are currently out of favour among editors, and the demand for case reports is much less than the supply. You now have to look around carefully for a journal that will take them. When you find one, use the **yellow marker test** to study the structure, which will vary from journal to journal. Think carefully about whether you have a suitable case – look in particular for a good message that will have immediate clinical relevance, such as the patient whose rash on the inside leg turned out to be a rare case of hepatitis M. Then approach this as you would approach any written work (*see* **process of writing**).

Chapters, writing of   *See* **books, writing of chapters in**.

Checking facts   This is important. Often it makes little substantive difference to the main thesis (Mr William Browne will have been sacked from his prestigious post regardless of the fact that you have left the 'e' off his name and have called him Mr Brown), but those who know will lose confidence in the rest of your writing – and gleefully tell others of your shortcomings. On the other hand, the nature of writing is such is that it is almost impossible to achieve 100% accuracy. So pay particular attention to things that matter: dosages, for instance, or names and titles. And don't become suicidal when the occasional error creeps in (*see* **law of late literals**).

Checklists   All kinds of people, from publishers to methodologists, produce checklists to use when writing papers and reviews. These are useful up to a point (or first 80 points!). But obsession with detail can obscure, or drive out, sensible **messages**. Good writing is not just a succession of facts put down in a plausible order (*see* **leaf shuffling**), but an interesting or important message, supported by evidence (*see* **truth**).

Christian names   This term is inappropriate in today's multicultural societies. Use 'first names'.

Citation index   *See* **impact factor**.

Clichés   The word comes from the French term for a printing block, and means a phrase that is reproduced so often that it is at best unoriginal, at worst tiresome. Clichés make splendid targets: for instance 'the focus on a fundamental shift in the culture of learning, leading to empowerment and a win-win situation'. However, some phrases, like 'ownership' and 'mission statement', have their own technical use among certain groups (*see* **jargon**). And some, like 'moving the goal posts' and 'gold standard' are a kind of shorthand that allow us to put across a familiar idea quickly and easily.

So what should the writer do? First, avoid choosing clichés that will cause your target reader (though not your **false feedback loop**) to ridicule you. Second, if you see a familiar phrase, ask yourself whether something more original would be a better choice. Don't feel you must get rid of them all: I have deliberately used several throughout this book. But don't over-egg the pudding.

Coaching. All too often people who write find that their only 'reward' is a mass of minor textual criticism. This is not normally considered the best way to develop and motivate people. Coaching is an alternative approach, based on the assumption that people do best at a task if they are allowed to get on with it themselves. Those with more writing experience should resist the temptation to give a mass of **'corrections'**, and instead offer support and encouragement. This approach is not necessarily taught in medical school.

Coaching can be of value at four different phases.

- *Strategy.* Many people feel that they should be writing (scientific papers, for instance) but aren't quite sure how. Encourage them to sit down and work out *why* they need to write. In the light of this, get them to commit to the *what* and the *when* (*see* **writing goals**).
- *Tactics.* Too many people launch themselves too quickly into a piece of writing. Encourage them to take time to **ruminate,** to set their own **brief** – and provide support at this early stage. Don't criticize, but probe with open-ended questions so that writers can develop their own ideas. Look for whether the writer has clearly defined the audience. Question how the writer will judge success (*see* **payoff**). Encourage research on the market as well as the topic being written about (*see* **evidence-based writing**). Set **deadlines.**
- *Execution.* Once the writing process has started, provide support and encouragement. Meet regularly to ensure that the deadlines are being met and, if not, work with the writer to find ways of getting the work moving again. Encourage **writers' support groups.** When (and if) the time comes for you to look at the manuscript, ask why you are being asked to read it – for silly mistakes, for instance, for major factual omissions or for potential political problems? Give **balanced feedback.** And give priority to keeping the copy moving: nothing demotivates more than to have work sitting in someone else's pending tray.
- *Reward.* Follow the example of successful sports coaches – and celebrate whenever you achieve your goals. Create a culture where winning – as defined by the writer in advance – is celebrated.

BOOKLIST: coaching

- *The coaching pocketbook,* by Ian Fleming and Allan JD Taylor, Alresford: Management Pocketbooks, 1998. Entertaining and versatile, part of an excellent series that also includes books on time management and personal development.
- *Writing your dissertation in 15 minutes a day,* by Joan Bolker, New York: Henry Holt, 1998. Ostensibly for those who are setting

out to write a thesis, this is perhaps even more useful for supervisors. Some interesting thoughts on setting up writers' groups.

- *Coaching writers: the essential guide for editors and reports*, by Roy Peter Clark and Don Fry, New York: St Martin's Press, 1992. An interesting book from two journalists in Florida with important lessons for those working with writers.

Co-authors

As a general rule, the greater the number of co-authors, the greater the problems. The manuscript over which you have been sweating for months is torn apart by others, who believe that they are failing if they are not pumping out as many criticisms as they can think of. The poor author is then left, manuscript and confidence in tatters, with a pile of alternative suggestions, many of them conflicting.

You will be pleased to know that there are some techniques that can ease the pain.

- *Arrange a meeting at the beginning of the writing process.* Agree who the co-authors will be, what they will do, and in which order they will appear on the manuscript (*see* **authorship**). Lay down deadlines, agree on the target journal and, more important still, get everyone to agree what the message will be (*see* **brief setting**).
- *Circulate the timetable among the co-authors.* Some people will always sit on a manuscript. If all co-authors have agreed on the deadlines, you have a lever which may help to move the laggards. Send co-authors regular updates of progress; this will enable everyone to identify those who are slowing the process down. Sometimes a bit of naming and shaming will help.
- *Involve your co-authors throughout the process.* Co-authors need to have a 'substantial intellectual involvement', but this does not necessarily mean detailed textual criticism once the work has been done. Far more important is the support and advice received as you are preparing the various drafts, and this is really the time you need sensible input from your colleagues. Keep them in touch with what you are doing, and encourage them to play the role of **coach** rather than critic.
- *Judge any comment from a co-author on whether it is more – or less – likely to get your paper published in your target journal.* One of the major problems at this stage is the mass of conflicting advice as each co-author proposes amendments on his or her notion of what makes a 'good' paper (*see* **Icarus fallacy**). The sensible way through this is to judge these comments on whether they are more

– or less – likely to increase the chances of publication (*see* **evidence-based writing**). Discuss those that are clearly counter productive (*see* **negotiating changes**).

- *Try to steer your co-authors into doing what you want them to do.* Instead of saying 'Please let me have your comments', which is an open invitation to be destructive, try, 'I enclose the draft of this article which, as you know, has been targeted at *The Lancet*. Can you let me know if you see any major omissions?' (If you have been keeping people involved (*see above*), then perhaps you can try: 'Can I assume that you are now happy for me to send it off?')

- *Don't take it personally.* Being criticized seems to be part of the publications game. Don't be demoralized. Keep reminding yourself that you are making progress and that this is one of the last major obstacles.

- *Do not be bullied into doing what you think is wrong.* Under no circumstances should you give in to pressure from co-authors to do anything that you think is morally wrong, such as make up patients who did not exist, or 'massage' the figures to make the work look better (*see* **scientific fraud**). This can be easier said than done, and if you are unlucky enough to be involved in such a situation, seek a wise head for immediate confidential advice.

If you survive your relationship with your co-authors, and you become published authors, celebrate. It will make all the aggravation and humiliation seem worthwhile – until the next time.

Colon   A punctuation mark that denotes a major pause that comes before an explanation or elaboration, as in, 'I am telling you something important in this section: it is how to use the colon appropriately'.

In US English usage it is common to have a capital letter after the colon ('He wanted three things: To visit every hospital in Poughkeepsie, write a book review for the *New Yorker*, and learn how to use chopsticks'). This is not the case in UK English, though your word processing package may not know this (*see* **semicolon; UK-US English**).

Colon dash(as in :-)   These are archaic, ugly and should not be used.

Commas

A punctuation mark that indicates a slight pause: 'He came and went' is different from 'he came, and went'. Commas are important, and can cause all kinds of howlers when omitted or wrongly placed, as in: 'The society is made up of those who experience difficulties in digestion of their relatives, and of other interested people'.

One of the big problems occurs when commas are used to make a separate and self-contained point, in which case they should always travel in pairs. 'The patients, who had demanded compensation rushed to their lawyers' is ambiguous. Does it mean that a group who had demanded compensation went to their lawyers while another group stayed put ('The patients who had demanded compensation rushed to their lawyers')? Or does it mean that a group of patients had rushed to their lawyers and all of them were demanding compensation ('The patients, who had demanded compensation, rushed to their lawyers)?

The use of commas in lists can cause confusion. This is because in **UK English** the comma is dropped before the 'and' ('stethoscopes, zebras and chairs'). This does not happen in **US English** ('stethoscopes, zebras, and chairs').

There is a fashion, particularly among medical journals, to be parsimonious with the comma. This can cause difficulties for the reader (*see* **grammar booklist**).

Commissioning

The success of most publications leans heavily on the quality of its contributors, so the ability to persuade good writers to contribute is an important skill (*see* **books, editing of**). Having an idea for an article is relatively easy; the hard thing is to find someone who will do it well (better than you, otherwise why bother?). Hardest of all is getting that person motivated.

Commissioning editors usually make the first contact by phone. If you are commissioning, have a clear idea of what you want: it is not helpful to give a long list of points that you wish the writer to include; instead describe what you want the article to achieve. Also discuss deadline, technical points (such as whether you want the article to be sent by e-mail) and payment or other reward.

Once you have agreement, write a follow-up letter, which should cover the following questions.

- *What kind of publication is it?* The writer should be clear about the goals of the publication – and about its audience. If you think the writer is unfamiliar with the publication, send one or two back copies.

- *Where in the publication will it go?* Knowing exactly where it will go will help the writer to do such basic things as write to length and ensure the right tone.
- *What do you want the article to do?* The writer needs a clear confirmation of the subject matter and broad intent, so that he or she can start to work out an appropriate message (*see* **brief setting**).
- *When do you need the copy?* You should have agreed this verbally, and it should be realistic for both of you. Make sure that it isn't so tight that failure to meet it will leave you in a completely impossible position.
- *How much you will pay (or any other reward)?* Nobody does anything for nothing so what will be in it for the writer? Spell out the reward in your letter.
- *Who will own the copyright?* This is a controversial issue nowadays and some editors may feel safer leaving this out and hoping for the best (*see* **copyright**).

If you have done your job, by the time the deadline comes you will have exactly what you want – or better. Now should come a frequently neglected step. Writers spend long and lonely hours, and usually crave reassurance it has been worthwhile. Many articles disappear into black holes, with authors getting feedback only when someone tells them they have seen the article in print. Commissioning editors, therefore, should always say thank you, by phone, e-mail, letter or in person.

If you decide that the article is not what you want, you can ask the writer to try again (in which case you have to be specific about the exact things he or she needs to do). Alternatively you can reject it, in which case you have a duty to return it as quickly as possible to the author, who may wish to submit it elsewhere (*see* **rejection**). You have a duty to be polite when rejecting an article, but you do not have to justify yourself at great length: sometimes things don't work out. In such cases you may wish to offer a slightly lower amount as a **kill fee**.

Committees   Keep them as far away as possible from the writing process. Anything written in committee usually ends up being written *for* the committee (or rather the powerful figures within it), not for the target audience (*see* **false feedback loop**).

Communication Getting a message across from one person to another. Writing something down does not guarantee this (*see* **effective writing**).

Communication theories Communication is a complicated business and there are all types of theories that take into account a wide range of factors influencing all those involved in the process, such as knowledge, context and motivation.

For **effective writing** as defined in this book, however, a basic reader-centred model will suffice. With this model, a writer sends a **message** that must be read – and understood – by the target reader. It may sound simple but it has some important implications. The first thing is that you are no longer writing for yourself or your colleagues (*see* **false feedback loop**). You can write in such a way to increase the chances of this happening (*see* **evidence-based writing**). You have a way of judging success: 'Did the target audience read it?' (*see* **effective writing**).

Competitions From time to time publications run writing competitions, often because they are an excellent way of finding new talent. If you want to break into these markets, watch out for them and enter. Even if you do not win, it will bring your writing to the attention of an editor, and this could be the start of a mutually beneficial relationship.

Compromise *See* **negotiating changes**.

Computers, writing on One of the great drawbacks of computers is that they can take much of the pain out of writing. This leads to two major problems. The first is enticing people to write too early (*see* **premature expostulation**). The second is that it allows people to sit and fiddle with what they have written. In such cases the solution is to print out a copy and do your **rewriting** on hard copy. This will at least allow you to have a sense of progress.

Computer screens If you cannot write a sentence without going back and fiddling with it, turn off your monitor (*see* **free writing**).

Concise writing   I find this a puzzling concept. Many people who come on my courses say they want to learn how to write more concisely. Yet these tend to be the ones who argue loudest in favour of long and flowery words and phrases. Perhaps concise writing is something they have been told they want, but don't actually want it (or value it) themselves (*see* **false feedback loop**).

Conference abstracts   Those with ambitions to travel and to advance their knowledge and careers need to master the art of the conference abstract. Unlike the **abstracts** published alongside a scientific paper, they stand alone, to be published in the conference abstract book. If you are lucky, they will earn you an invitation to produce a poster, or present a paper.

Approach conference abstracts as you would any other writing task (*see* **process of writing**). In particular research carefully what the organizers want: this means looking carefully through all the advance material you can get hold of. It also means looking at the material from last year's conference. Study the **structure** of previous abstracts. Look also at the topics dealt with in the past; try to find something that will develop these ideas and discussions.

Conference reports   Those who attend conferences are often asked by those who don't to 'write it up'. This sounds a straight-forward task, but isn't. The main problem is that these conferences churn out thousands (if not millions) of words; the writer's task is to cut them down to about 1000 and arrange them in a way that will attract the uncommitted reader. You clearly cannot cover everything and everyone, so these reports are neither a précis nor a set of **minutes**.

Avoid clinging to the order of the conference proceedings ('In the early afternoon we heard an excellent presentation on sentence construction before moving on to the future of the paragraph after tea ...'). Avoid also using the shape of a scientific article (*see* **IMRAD structure**). Prefer the **feature article** structure: from all the informa-tion you will have collected, formulate a message and then choose to put in only the information that will support and elaborate that message.

- *Get a good brief from the start.* Make sure you get detailed informa-tion from whoever asks you to write the report (*see* **commis-sioning**). Which publication and what kind of audience? What

27

format? Is there an example of the kind of conference report they like (and perhaps one they don't)?

- *At the conference, just soak up the information.* Don't just listen to the proceedings, but look at notice boards, exhibitions and anything else that takes your fancy. These could provide detail and colour to lift your report out of the mundane. At the same time try to make sense of it all. What's new? What's interesting? What would the readers like to hear about?

- *After the conference, decide on a message.* Lack of data is rarely the problem; the difficulty is how to order it. As with all types of writing, start with the basics: construct a 12 word message from the conference, then go through the usual stages (*see* **process of writing**).

- *Don't be afraid to leave things out.* This is not a shopping list but a brief account. What some might call bias is necessary selection; don't be afraid to do it.

Conferences
Gatherings of the professional tribes, usually at someone else's expense. A great way of travelling to foreign parts (*see* **conference abstracts**).

Conflict of interest
Many travel articles are followed by a brief statement stating whether their tickets have been paid for, and if so by whom. Similarly, many papers in scientific journals make it clear if the work has been supported by the pharmaceutical company whose product is being tested.

The point is that readers have the right to assume that the views expressed in an article are honestly held, and are not being expressed for other reasons, such as an expenses-paid trip to Monte Carlo. If publications are not trusted, they lose their usefulness (*see* **Pravda effect**). If there is any reason for anyone to suppose that bias could take place, then it must be declared. Failure to do so looks suspicious.

Confusing pairs
Some words are troublesome because they sound the same as other words (*see* **homophones**); others give trouble because they are confused with other words that sound different – but not too different. Here is a sample:

- *affect* and *effect*: (1) to influence, and (2) to accomplish,
- *alleviate* and *elevate*: (1) to lessen, and (2) to raise or increase,

- *continual* and *continuous*: (1) very often, and (2) unbroken,
- *flaunt and flout*: (1) to display ostentatiously, and (2) to display contempt for (the law etc.),
- *prescribe* and *proscribe*: (1) to suggest a course of action, (2) to forbid,
- *prostrate* and *prostate*. (1) lying down, and (2) male gland.

Controversy   Editors realize that there is nothing better for readership than a good row. So they welcome controversy, up to a point (*see* **lawyers**).

Copy   Journalists' term for a piece of writing, as in 'Where's the bloody copy?'.

Copy-editors   People used by book publishers (mainly) to put text into house style, correct grammar and spelling, and to point out infelicities (such as, in this case, my failure in the first draft to give copy-editors an entry of their own). They can perform invaluable services. *See also* **technical editors; subeditors**.

Copyright   This establishes the creator of a piece of original work and protects authors against others stealing the idea or making money out of copying it, often badly. There are two ways in which it affects authors.

First, you must seek permission if you want to use substantial pieces of text, charts or tables from another article. The precise definition of the word 'substantial' keeps many lawyers and their family in luxury, so if in doubt, pass the buck swiftly to your publisher. Most publishers ask authors to assign the copyright to them, so this task is fairly straightforward.

Then there is the question of how authors, particularly those working on their own, can ensure that they, and not their publisher, will make the money their brilliance deserves. This has always been difficult, and the new freedoms of the **World Wide Web** will make it more so. I suspect that this is one of those areas where the amount of effort (and loss of goodwill) is usually outweighed by the actual amount of money involved. The simple answer is that, if your idea is

29

that good, then you should immediately get yourself an **agent**, who can carry out these unpopular arguments on your behalf.

Correcting the work of others   We often use the word 'corrections' to describe the marks that other people have put over what we have written. In fact they are usually changes, and not corrections (*see* **balanced feedback**).

Corrections   Publishing anything is a complicated business, and mistakes are inevitable (*see* **law of late literals**). Editors clearly have a duty to their readers to correct information that has been proved to be wrong. In some cases, this is relatively trivial: 'In yesterday's obituary we said that John Brown-Green died in a car accident in Barnes. In fact it was in East Sheen.' In other cases, such as publishing an incorrect dose, it could be a matter of life and death (*see* **proofreading**).

Coughing   The habit of starting a piece of writing with some weak words ('It is interesting to note that ...', 'Some observers have noted ...') that could be moved to the end of the sentence or even cut out altogether. These can be identified quite easily with the **first six words test**. However, with letters, the convention is to start with a polite cough in the first sentence: 'Thank you so much for your kind letter ...' or, 'It was so nice to meet you last Saturday'.

Court action   Best to avoid (*see* **lawyers; libel**).

Covering letter   Presentation is an important part of the battle to impress an **editor**, and the covering letter offers an excellent opportunity to make a good impression from the start. In particular you will have the opportunity to establish three things.
- *Who you are.* This comes partly from your name and title at the bottom of the letter, but also from a range of other things – for instance, the formal stationery on which the letter is written; the typeface that is chosen and the way it is presented; written cues, such as, 'our team has already published in your journal'; and even the style (friendly, pompous, illiterate?) in which you phrase

the letter. If you are submitting to magazines and newspapers for the first time, you may wish to enclose some cuttings of previous articles you have had published in similar publications.

- *What you are offering.* Avoid the formulaic 'Enclosed please find herewith my paper *Letters to the editor: a multicentre double-blind trial.*' This is dull (most journal titles are dull). Sell your **message**: 'I enclose a copy of our paper which proves for the first time that writing covering letters of more than 200 words increases dramatically the chance of being published.' Putting the title at the top of the letter, as a heading, will give you the best of both worlds.

- *Why the editor will benefit from publishing what you have written.* The final paragraph of your letter gives you an opportunity to sell. Do so gently. Avoid veiled threats ('I am a member of the disciplinary committee of the Royal College of Medical Communicators'), bribes ('I hope that you will be our guest at our next congress in Rio de Janeiro') and sycophantic appeals ('I am a regular reader of your excellent journal'). But you may wish to drop in the fact that your research gives the next step in a series of findings published by the journal, or that it genuinely adds to the debate on an important topic. If you feel brave, try humour ('Our finding is so important and your journal so well-read that they belong to one another') but it can be a dangerous game to play.

With most journals, the covering letter to the editor will also have a number of formal requirements. Many journals, for instance, require all co-authors to sign. Carefully read the **Instructions to Authors** to see what is required.

Editors of course will swear that they are never influenced by such things. But then they would, wouldn't they?

Crap   A useful term in certain circles to describe a piece of writing that does not work. This does not necessarily mean that the writer is a failure, though it does suggest that he or she should go back and do some more work (*see* **process of writing**). Do not use this term in front of the author (*see* **balanced feedback**).

Creativity   In general we can favour this, but use it in the way you select and organize your information – and not to indulge in extravagant ways of expressing yourself.

Criteria of good writing   Rarely shared and agreed (*see* **effective writing**).

Criticism   An important part of the writing process. It should be constructive, but rarely is (*see* **balanced feedback**).

Cutting things out   This is inevitable. But it takes up a lot of time and you should, within reason, be producing first drafts of roughly the right length. If you find that you are regularly having to cut out large chunks of text, you might wish to re-examine the way you write (*see* **leaf shuffling**).

CV   Producing CVs involves a difficult balancing act: we need to produce a short account of our life that will be flashy enough to sell us above the heads of dozens, perhaps hundreds, of rivals – without laying ourselves open to the shameful crime of self-promotion. The important thing to remember is that CVs are not an all-inclusive description of our entire life and times, but a tool to get us on the shortlist.

- *Keep updating the information.* Regular updates will ensure that you always have on hand the raw material needed to produce high quality CVs quickly. They will encourage you to keep reviewing what you have done – and what you still need to do (*see* **goal setting**).
- *Do some market research.* Try to see what others are currently producing, either by asking around or, perhaps, by volunteering to sit on a selection committee yourself. Compare the CVs of those who have been shortlisted with those who have not, not just in terms of what information they include, but also in terms of how they are presented. Don't buck the accepted conventions: a young doctor of my acquaintance recently had a talented designer friend 'modernize' her CV; she got no interviews. When she returned to the more conventional format, the interview offers started to return (*see* **marketing**).
- *Match the CV to the job.* With word processors there is no excuse for not tailoring each CV for each job. Ask yourself: what are they looking for? You may wish to give something a little more prominence or cut out something else; it will take only a few minutes.
- *Keep it factual.* Avoid vague terms ('prolific author') and keep to the information (published papers in 23 journals, including seven

in the *NEJM* and two in *The Lancet*) (*see* **nouns**). Make sure that there are no errors of fact: if you describe your stay at St Ann's Hospital there is bound to be someone there who knows that it is really St Anne's.

- *Don't raise unanswered questions.* The gap of two years when you cooked hamburgers in a bar in Viareggio may have no direct relevance to your subsequent career, but you may need to explain why there is a two-year gap. If not, people may jump to uncharitable conclusions, such as a two-year prison sentence. (If you have had a two-year prison sentence, then you may need to take expert advice on how to handle this.)

- *Pay attention to outside interests.* Many interviewers say that these are unimportant; I don't believe them. Most CVs contain the same kind of information about careers, perhaps with the odd prize or publication thrown in, or appointments at more prestigious institutions. This means that the section on 'outside interests' may be your best chance of putting yourself above the crowd. You need more than 'walking, reading, eating in restaurants and going to the cinema'. If you can't think of anything, develop some interests – such as playing rugby against or for the All Blacks, appearing as an extra in films, or teaching young offenders how to cook. Be prepared to talk about these in the interview.

- *Present your CV carefully.* Choose one or two standard **typefaces** and avoid **polyfontophilia**. Keep the type size large (12 point is the convention), and under no circumstances reduce the type size to fit in all the words; if you have too many, cut some out, which by definition means that you are improving the product. Keep sensible margins, so that the text is framed within white space, giving a sense of organization. Send off a decent copy, not the photocopy of the photocopy.

- *Imagine yourself one of the selectors.* They will be seeing dozens of these. What is in yours that will get you shortlisted?

The one good thing about CVs is that you will have no difficulty in judging quality. If they are consistently getting you shortlisted, then they are good enough. If you are not getting the jobs, however, you may have to brush up on your interview technique.

Dangling modifiers   This is the error made when a phrase is misplaced, away from the word it relates to. As in (from an earlier draft of this book): 'Derived from a French word that described the twittering of birds, the famous war correspondent Russell used the word 'jargon' in a different sense ...'. That is untrue: the famous war correspondent was a product of the union of Mr and Mrs Russell, and not of a French word. The error seems to be more common among those who have had a **Latin education**.

Dashes   A useful piece of **punctuation**. A pair can act in the same way as a pair of commas (The patient, who appeared smartly dressed – with a collar and tie and a yellow socks – at the clinic, was clearly very ill'), or for indicating a pause that is slightly more dramatic than that afforded by a colon: 'He was very smartly dressed – with a collar and tie, no less'). Don't over-use them.

Data junkies   Those who are obsessed with accumulating all manner of data for their writing, thereby ensuring that the whole thing becomes not only unreadable but also unfinished. It is difficult to convince such people that they are wasting everyone's time, including their own (*see* **leaf shuffling; writer's block**).

Deadlines   Some treat these as abstract notions, put down for the convenience of editors. In fact publications would cease to exist without deadlines. They ensure that those putting together the publication are able to cope with the many different and complex sequences of tasks needed. It gives editors a good chance of producing a journal-type publication regularly, which in turn means that readers are more likely to get into the habit of reading it.

Some people break deadlines all the time, often by the same amount of time on each occasion. This tends to be either a personal statement ('I am more important than you, so don't push me around') or a problem in technique (such as failing to allow enough time for others to have their input). If you are an editor, your duty is clear: if you start to allow people to break deadlines you will be in trouble, so be firm – and have an alternative up your sleeve so that you will be able to fill the pages. You will rarely have to do this more than once: nothing changes writers' attitudes to deadlines as quickly as the realization that they won't be published if they flout them.

In fact successful writers realize that deadlines have uses for them also, and those who don't have them imposed by others usually impose them on themselves. Deadlines provide a target. They also define the point beyond which writers will stop fiddling (*see* **perfection**).

Things tend to go wrong when we set deadlines that are too vague. Writing is not one task but several – in other words **project management**. The trick is to lay out in advance, preferably in a diary, the various stages that you will have to go through. Be sensible in your projections (*see* **time management**) and allow plenty of time for rewriting (*see* **process of writing**).

Declarative titles   These are titles with a verb in them. Thus: 'Acute application of NGF increases the firing rate of aged rat basal forebrain neurons.' The alternative is an 'indicative' title, which as its name suggests, indicates what the authors looked at, but doesn't give away what they found: 'Expression of glutamate transporters in rat optic nerve oligodendrocytes'.

There is widespread agreement among newspaper and magazine journalists, who have access to detailed market research on how people read, that putting a verb in a headline (i.e. making it declarative) will increase dramatically the chances of attracting uncommitted readers. Even if they don't read the article, they will have seen the main message. Yet many journal editors remain passionately attached to the indicative title.

Where does this leave the writer? Fortunately there is a clear answer: look in your target journal and follow the style you see there (*see* **evidence-based writing**). As a general rule, the US journals are more likely to use the declaratory style while some UK journals, led by the *BMJ*, prefer two strings of nouns, linked by a **colon**.

Decorated municipal gothic   Defined by the writer and broadcaster Michael O'Donnell as 'a prose style that evolves when writers eschew simple words that might express their ideas in a neat and palatable form and use instead language they believe adds dignity, scientific worth, or even grandeur to their utterance, as in: "This vehicle is being utilized for highway cleansing purposes" or (using a medical example) "alimentation was maintained" (*A Sceptic's Medical Dictionary*, Michael O'Donnell, London: BMJ Books, 1997, p. 48).

The genre persists, particularly in papers submitted to committees, as in this example: 'The strategy represents "extra effort" and fresh focus on the part of the main partners to address the key priorities identified. It will not lead to a diminution of existing core service provision.' English translation: 'Our new strategy will not harm existing services' (*see* **flabby phrases; gravitas; putting on the posh overcoat; style [1]**).

Defamation   The act of damaging someone's reputation with words to such an extent that he or she is awarded damages in court. It can be spoken (**slander**) or written (**libel**). The classic definitions include exposing someone to 'hatred, ridicule and contempt', or 'lowering them in the estimation of right-thinking members of society generally'. The allegation has to be 'published' to a third party, in a publication for instance, or a letter that a secretary opens.

Of the available defences, the following two seem fairly easy to understand (though be warned, many lawyers have become exceedingly rich discussing their exact meanings and implications).

- *Truth.* You have to be able to prove that, for instance, the 'commie bastard' is a paid-up member of the party and that his mother never married, or that the 'deadly doctor' has clearly killed large numbers of patients administering 500 mg when the label clearly said 5 mg.
- *Privilege.* If someone makes an allegation about another in court or in parliament, it is 'protected by privilege'; in other words, the normal laws of defamation would not apply. However, repeat the statement later, and you could well face a defamation action.

The problem with these defences is that they take huge amounts of time to assemble. So the best rule is: *if in doubt, leave it out.*

For most readers of this book, the risk of libelling someone should not be high. But take care when writing book reviews and even refereeing papers. As a general rule you can say someone has done bad work (we all do that from time to time), but you can't say that they are incompetent or, even worse, dishonest. 'Professor Beychevelle's study on the benefits of claret is flawed' is fine. 'Professor Beychevelle's study on the benefits of claret is doubtless influenced by the fact that his chair is funded by the Association of Claret Growers' is not – there is a clear implication that he has changed the data to suit the sponsors.

What happens if you suspect fraud in a paper that you are asked to review? This is a difficult one, and I suspect the best solution is to ring the editor yourself – on a land-line – and put nothing in writing.

If you have written something that someone claims is libelling him or her, act with great caution. Contact the editor at once: most publications have libel insurance and they will immediately seek legal advice on your (and now their) behalf. Trying to sort it out yourself will almost certainly make things worse.

BOOKLIST: legal problems

- *McNae's Essential law for journalists*, London: Butterworths, 1999. For those who are really interested, this is the standard book for journalists. It is constantly being updated.

Defensive writing   Writing that is drafted to avoid trouble, such as embarrassment in open court, rather than to put a message across. This is a type of **political writing**; don't confuse it with **effective writing**.

Demotivation   When it comes to the writing of scientific papers, this seems to have been elevated to an art form. All the mechanisms of 'support' seem set to criticize writers, not support them. Yet there are valuable techniques, such as **coaching, balanced feedback** and **evidence-based writing**.

Design   Should be kept for the professionals. **Layout** you can do.

Desks   Keep them uncluttered; otherwise you may be unable to resist the temptation to stop writing and start fiddling.

Dictating machines   Some feel that it is cheating to use them, but they are extremely useful. They are fast, they encourage us to use a speaking vocabulary rather than a posh writing one (*see* **pub test**) and they make it difficult for us to keep track of what we have said so that we plough on rather than fiddle around with what we have just said. All this helps us to get down the all-important **first draft.**

The disadvantage is that we can get carried away with the sound of our own voice and our own brilliance. We can end up somewhere totally unexpected and quite useless. And we need someone to transcribe what we have done.

There are two precautions to take: (1) make sure you are entirely clear what you are saying (*see* **brief setting**) and (2) leave plenty of time for **rewriting**. However much you enjoyed speaking at the time, there will certainly be some tidying up to do.

The development of voice recognition computers may make dictating machines redundant. Within a few years we could all be dictating our first draft straight onto our personal computer, which no doubt will bring up a whole range of new problems.

Doctors   They are highly trained in medical matters; they are not usually highly trained in writing matters.

Double negatives   These are not uncommon. Alas, they are equally not inconducive to incomprehension. Thus we cannot exclude them from being considered harmless.

Draft   *See* **first draft**.

Duplicate publication   Magazines and newspapers compete against each other, and therefore consider it quite wrong for an author to offer the same article to more than one publication at a time. However, in these markets it is usually considered acceptable to write a similar article for a non-competing market (a newspaper for doctors and a journal for nurses, for instance). To avoid inadvertently biting the hand that you are asking to feed you, it makes sense to tell both editors what you are doing. If you later want to revisit the topic, and write it for a publication in the same market, but in a substantially different way, then this is considered acceptable; in fact, from a freelance's point of view, it is good practice.

When it comes to writing for journals, the matter gets rather more complicated. Journal editors feel aggrieved if they publish an article that has appeared elsewhere. Also, since publication is now used as a key performance indicator (*see* **CV**), many people feel that it is cheating to get two sets of points for one piece of work (*see also* **salami publication**).

There is a clear solution for writers: under no circumstances should you send the same article to more than one editor at a time, nor should you revamp a published original scientific article and send it to another journal. If in any doubt, speak to the editor.

There is a trickier issue, which is whether authors can write the same – or a similar – scientific article in two different languages. It seems reasonable that someone who has written an interesting article in one language should be allowed to communicate to those who speak (only) another. However, the author should make it absolutely clear what is being done: he or she should refer to the previous paper, thereby putting everything in the open and enabling the editor to make a decision in full view of the facts. Failure to do so is **scientific fraud**.

Ear   A useful tool for judging whether a piece of writing works. This is why many people find it useful to read aloud (preferably to themselves, quietly) what they have written.

Easy reading   Something we all value, unless we happen to be doing the writing at the time (*see* **effective writing**).

Editing   *See* **books, editing of; copy-editor; editor; macro-editing; micro-editing; subeditor; technical editor.**

Editor   This is the person at the centre of a publication, who is responsible for what is and what is not published, and who therefore defines the publication's 'soul'. It is a key position, and editors find themselves co-ordinating a web of activities:
- ensuring that the publication has enough funds to keep publishing;
- gathering and presenting material;

- setting deadlines and ensuring that they are met;
- making sure that readers receive their copies, and so on.

They have to juggle a range of competing interests, particularly those of proprietors, readers, authors and the 'general good'.

There can be confusion here, because the verb 'to edit' has another meaning, which is to take a submitted article, and improve it. This is the task done by a **copy-editor, subeditor** or **technical editor**. Sometimes, particularly on small publications or newsletters, the same person will be editor and subeditor, but there is a clear difference between the two roles.

Being an editor of (as opposed to for) an 'ongoing publication' is a time-consuming task. Before you accept the honour, consider the following advice.

- *Don't start unless you are absolutely clear what your role is to be.* Do not accept responsibility without power. Find out where the limits of your power will be – to whom will you report and under what circumstances can you be fired? This is particularly important if you are being appointed by a professional (as opposed to a commercial) organization (*see* **editorial freedom, editorial integrity**).

- *Maintain clear lines of communication with your employers.* Find out what they want from you, and be sure to let them know when you achieve it. If you anticipate trouble, warn them. And remember to massage their egos (*see* **managing upwards**).

- *Define your readership precisely – and serve it obsessively.* Publications work if they meet the needs of a definable group of people – the readership. One of the first tasks of the editor is to decide in his or her mind what this group is – and what distinguishes them from other groups. Once these people are defined, the task is to keep them faithful. If you fail to define your readers, or try to please those who aren't readers (*see* **false feedback loop**), or try to reconcile irreconcilable groups of potential readers, then you could be in trouble.

- *Have a clear view of what you are trying to do.* A large part of the job consists of deciding what goes in and where, and you must make these decisions rationally. To do this, you need to have a clear idea of (a) where your publication is going, (b) how you will get there, and (c) how you will know when you do. Make sure all those involved (from owners to readers to contributors) know all this (*see* **mission**).

- *Don't be afraid to turn things down.* Unless you reject contributions, you are working as a clerical assistant, not an editor. That doesn't mean that you can ignore basic principles of courtesy, like thanking people for what they have done (*see* **commissioning**).

- *Form a team and motivate its members.* Unless you have contributions from others, you are writing a pamphlet, not editing a publication. Seek out people who will contribute their energies and diverse talents. The key is motivation – enthusing them with your view of the future and helping them to share in the rewards. These could be vulgar financial ones – or something less tangible such as job satisfaction, praise, and a feeling of teamwork.
- *Don't have delusions of grandeur.* Keep everything in perspective. People may treat you as a very important person, but that's mainly so that you can be nice to them. Watch how quickly the invitations dry up when you leave your post.
- *Keep trust with your readers.* Readers nowadays are unlikely to expect that your publication consists solely of the **Truth**, but they do have the right to assume that the articles are honestly written, and that they have been chosen on merit and not because money or some other favours have secretly changed hands.

If approached with care and proper planning (*see* **time management**), the role of editor will help you to forge new friendships, put you in touch with exciting developments, involve you in some challenging decisions, expose you to challenging ideas and force you to learn new skills. It may even allow you to do a little bit of good in the world, but don't count on it.

Editor, dealing successfully with

The writer–editor relationship is like the patient–doctor relationship: you are highly dependent on someone else's goodwill. Make sure that you do not become a heartsink writer by following these guidelines.

- *Give editors what they want.* Good contributors will solve problems, not cause them. In particular they will solve the editor's need to fill blank pages with material that will interest their readers. If you can do this, you will be made welcome.
- *Research your market thoroughly.* One of the most common reasons why editors reject articles is that they are not right for their publication. They find this tiresome because, in most instances, the writers could and should have been able to work this out for themselves. Look at the various sections in the publication, and the type of writing in each (*see* **evidence-based writing**). Look also for any **Instructions to Authors,** and follow them to the letter. If you still have any questions or doubts, then ring up the publication.

- *Ask yourself why the editor should trust you.* If you are not known at the publication, make sure that you establish your identity in a way that can be easily checked. Write a covering letter. If you have been published already, enclose a few cuttings. Don't expect them to be read, but your chances of being published in the *Little Snodgrass Gazette* won't be harmed by a byline or two in *The Times* or even the *British Medical Journal*.
- *Respect the editor's decision.* Writing is a personal and lonely activity, and this can fool writers into believing that their work is better than it is. Trust the editor's judgement: after all making decisions is what editors are paid to do. Be careful about arguing: what you are really saying is that in your opinion the editor is unfit to edit. This is unlikely to make him or her change their mind (*see* **rejection**).
- *Don't quibble about pay.* Money can be very destructive in a relationship, so take care. The main thing is getting published, and then getting published again. Arguing that you should have been paid £120 not £110 will not help in the pursuit of this task; it will probably leave a rather sour taste in the mouth of a formerly supportive (and possibly less well paid) editor.
- *Don't get it wrong.* Editors have to take a leap of faith when deciding whether to publish. Don't betray that trust by submitting articles that have been sloppily researched (*see* **checking facts**).

Editorial boards   Many journals have long lists of eminent people from all over the world who make up their editorial board. This is useful marketing: being able to drop the names of all these dignitaries adds prestige. It also helps to attract contributions, not only from members of the board but from their colleagues and friends.

It's fine at this level, when those given this honour have so many other things to do that they have little time left over for interfering. But for smaller publications, particularly newsletters, it can be a dangerous model to follow. Some organizations favour them at this level because they believe that they spread the load (and make sure no one gets too important). Unfortunately, these committees (for that is what they are) tend to increase the editor's workload as they dream up more and more ideas, but melt away when it comes to implementing them. They also threaten to divert the publication from serving the needs of readers to serving the needs of the board members.

For those still considering an editorial board, here are some sensible questions.

- *What will be the benefits of an editorial board?* Committees can be expensive in time and money. They can also be unpredictable and irrational. Go ahead only if you think these disadvantages will be outweighed by the advantages – such as widening the network of supporters, providing political back-up, or adding prestige and credibility.
- *Is their task tightly defined?* If you decide to go ahead, have a clear view of what the role of the committee should be. Make it clear what power they will have and what duties they will perform.
- *Does the agenda reflect this role?* Do you want the board to give ideas, or do you want them to 'review' your last issue (which will probably add little to anything other than your own discomfort)?
- *Have you prepared thoroughly?* Meetings such as this can suddenly have a collective rush of blood to the head, and charge off in a direction that is as dangerous as it is unexpected. Take time to plan, producing written reports to back up your proposals and undertaking personal lobbying on the more important issues.
- *What's in it for them?* Altruism is a rare commodity, so people who sit on such committees tend to want something in return. Sometimes you will get away with giving them a bland meeting and an exciting meal (better than the other way round). But not always.

Editorial freedom   Not a useful concept. Unless editors are also owner-publishers, they are inevitably responsible to a more powerful individual or organization. A more useful concept is that of **editorial integrity**.

Editorial integrity   Clearly editors are unable to act completely freely. They have legal constraints (though it is part of their role to push against these). They have responsibilities to readers to publish material that is accurate and true, as far as is reasonably possible. Finally, they have a responsibility towards the owners (or owner) who fund the publication, and have a right to expect that it does not actively oppose their interests.

The solution is two-fold. An editor must have the right to edit, in other words have the last word on what is or is not published. At the same time, the owners have the right to change editors if they feel he or she has taken the wrong decisions. Editing therefore becomes the art of the possible, and one of the main tasks is to ensure that he or she can carry out the actions needed to fulfil their vision. This involves the key skill of **managing upwards**, which is not taught in medical schools.

Editorial material   The generic term for written material in a publication. This distinguishes it from **advertising**. Mixing the two produces the unsatisfactory and confusing mess known as **advertorial**.

Editorials   A piece of writing, displayed in a prominent position, that expresses a strong view on a matter of importance to a publication's readers. They are also called leading articles or leaders. Many newspapers, magazines and journals have these as unsigned articles, so that the whole weight of the publication can go behind it. Writing them is considered to be one of the more elevated tasks and those writing them are allowed to be unusually pompous.

Some medical journals have moved away from this tradition of anonymous comment towards signed editorials, which themselves seem to be moving towards state-of-the-subject reviews (*see* **review articles**). In these, the opinion clearly belongs to those who wrote and signed them.

If you are invited to write an editorial, analyse carefully the type of product that is expected. Look through several in the target publication and identify in particular the **structure** and the **language**.

Effective writing   Defining this is one of the most important issues in this book. Unfortunately, many people are vague about what they consider to be good writing, and define it in subjective terms: 'I know it when I see it. It sort of flows. And it's elegant' (*see* **style**).

I favour a more practical definition: *effective writing achieves the purpose we set it*. Effective writing does not set out to be obscure and misunderstood (*see* **political writing**), nor is it written to satisfy some urge within the writer (*see* **great writers**). It is not an art form but a tool, and the way to measure it is to set out in advance what you want to do. This then becomes the standard you can measure it against.

For instance, you can consider an article a 'good' one when it is accepted for publication in your target journal (waiting for praise is likely to disappoint). Consider a report successful when your preferred recommendations get accepted. Be satisfied with a letter if the recipient comes back for more information, or (under different circumstances) does not come back for more information. A leaflet appealing for blood donors can be considered a success when the target number of donors appears.

The principle is that writing is your servant, not your master. If you define in advance what you want your writing to do, you can also define in advance how to measure it. Failure to do this can lead to confusion and depression as you start to believe those who tell you, for all kinds or reasons and with no real evidence, that your writing is poor (*see* **PIANO**).

Effort   What is needed to turn the **first draft** into something that the reader will look at, continue to read, understand and act upon. Sadly there is no alternative to this, and don't believe those who tell you otherwise.

Electives   Medical students find these exciting things to do, and not surprisingly many of them come back wanting to write about them. Unfortunately this means that it's hard to find a market for them. To stand a chance of being published, they must contain an original message. This means more than finding an exotic destination (*see* **travel writing**).

Electronic publishing   Written communications are in the middle of a revolution which is making, and will continue to make, dramatic changes to the way we read and write. In the old days (though not that long ago – the pace of change is so fast), if we wanted to distribute what we had written, we reproduced it on paper and provided each reader with a copy. Now the situation has been turned on its head. With the global network of interlinking computers (*see* **World Wide Web**), producing more copies for more people requires little extra cost.

This has brought some major opportunities, particularly to the world of scientific publishing. Papers can now be published much faster, and the process of **peer review** can take place publicly, even as the paper is being formed, on the **World Wide Web**. The balance between supply and demand will change, so that any paper considered of adequate quality by the reviewers can now be published.

The implications are great. There will be migration towards the higher status journals, and those lower down the scale will have difficulty finding original papers. Even the prestigious journals may start to move towards a secondary role – not publishing original papers, but giving information and summaries about those they have published on their Web sites. Journals will move away from their modern role of validating science and defining hierarchies, and back towards their original role of informing readers about significant new developments.

There are still many fundamental questions still left unanswered. How will publishers make money from electronic publishing? Will there be a role for traditional publishers, or will the task of publishing original papers be taken over by other organizations? How will we find our way around, or will we all start to suffer from information overload? Most important of all, what will happen if the power goes off?

E-mails, writing of   One of the curious things about e-mails is that, even in the workplace, many of them still retain a freshness that has long since disappeared from other types of writing (*see* **putting on the posh overcoat**). I suspect that this is because people generally write to a named person, which means that they have a clear definition of the **target audience**. E-mails are sent immediately, so there is no time for the **false feedback loop** to come into effect.

No doubt this will change, and some e-mails will start to be as boring as other types of writing. Meanwhile, enjoy.

Embargo   A notice put on a press release requesting that publication of the news is delayed until a certain date and time. This system is useful when the **press release** is linked to an event, like the budget speech or the Queen's list of honours, because it allows those working in the media to prepare in advance and come up with well-researched reports as soon as the event has taken place. Some public relations advisers overdo it, putting on artificial embargoes: these are likely to be broken.

Emphasis   Many people embark on a false and gimmicky quest to give emphasis. Thus they will put words in CAPITAL LETTERS, or in **bold type** or in *italics*. This may work in small doses: it *can* be effective to use italics to emphasize one word, as here, *but if you use it for more than a word or two it becomes difficult to read, according to a number of studies* (*see* **research on writing**). Putting something into a box is also a bad solution: the evidence suggests that people tend to notice boxes, but ignore what goes in them.

The best solution is to order your words in such a way that the natural cadences will emphasize the words and phrases you wish to emphasize. We read in certain ways, which gives us key positions to exploit, in particular the start and the end of a sentence, paragraph or piece of writing. If you want to emphasize a single word, put it at the end of the sentence. If you want to emphasize a sentence, place it at the beginning or end of your writing (*see* **first sentence; final sentence**).

Endings *See* **final sentence.**

English English is not one language, but several, all of which are developing in different ways. Use the version that is most appropriate to your target audience (*see* **evidence-based writing**). Don't be afraid to enlist the help of someone who is familiar with the particular brand of English you choose.

English teachers They have a lot to answer for. Behind many writers lurks a figure from their youth, who clearly traumatized them, destroying their confidence and instilling into them false rules about the use of 'and' and split infinitives. It is important for those traumatized in this way to realize that they have moved on and should no longer be writing to please their teachers (*see* **audience; false feedback loop**).

Enthusiasm Be wary of those who wax lyrical about how much they enjoy writing; most rational people hate it. Those who argue otherwise are either fooling themselves (and boring their audiences), or lying.

Evidence-based writing My concept of 'evidence-based writing' is simple. If you have defined carefully your target **audience,**

then the type of writing you need is the type of writing that has worked for that audience in the past. If writing for a journal, follow the style of that journal; if writing for a newspaper, follow the style of that newspaper; if writing a report for a committee, then follow the style of reports that have been previously accepted. And so on.

This puts writing on a rational basis. Instead of arguing endlessly whether to use **jargon,** or **pompous initial capitals,** or **split infinitives,** or the **passive voice,** look at the evidence of what your target audience prefers. This approach will save hours of argument and stress (*see* **negotiating changes**).

Examinations

Many otherwise intelligent professionals still approach writing as if they have to 'get it right' first time. This is probably because much of their writing has been dominated by the unnatural act of sitting examinations – taking a couple of hours to regurgitate previously memorized information. We all need to move on: treat writing not as a measure of goodness or cleverness or niceness, but as a powerful tool of communication (*see* **effective writing**).

Exclamation marks

Most people insist that they should be used only to signal an exclamation and not to signal a weak joke. After many years repeating this advice (but ignoring it in my own writing!), I think the time has come to change positions: they can be very useful to signal a weak joke. But don't overdo it.

Executive summary

A shortened version of a long and boring **report,** but a great opportunity to do some **effective writing,** and much, much more than an abstract tacked on at the last minute because that's the way it's done.

The purpose of writing reports is to make recommendations and provide evidence in favour of implementing them. They follow certain conventions – they are lengthy, full of data, and written in a formal 'professional' language. The goal of the executive summary, on the other hand, is to sell the recommendations to the busy decision-makers. It should be shorter (rarely more than a single page), written in a more accessible language (*see* **readability scores**), and use the more reader-friendly **inverted triangle** structure.

This reiterates one of the recurrent themes of this book: if you want to write successfully for two different audiences you need two different pieces of writing.

Facts, checking   *See* **checking of facts**

Failure, fear of   A major reason why people don't write (*see* **process of writing**).

Fairness   Readers have a right to expect that an article has been selected for publication because the editor has decided that publication is in the audience's interest. Contributors and authors have a right to be dealt with promptly and openly. Editors have a right to be treated fairly by contributors and authors, who should respect an editor's right to decide which of several acceptable submissions should be published (*see* **rejection**).

False feedback loop   One of the most dangerous parts of writing comes when we give what we have written to others for informal advice or formal approval. Unless handled carefully (*see* **balanced feedback**), this can become an extremely demotivating stage. More importantly, changes made now may destroy much of the good work already done. This is not because these people are out to get us, but because they are all working to their own agendas.

I describe this as the 'false feedback loop': it is the pressure from those commenting on a piece of writing to have it changed, so that it meets their purposes rather than those of the target audience. This explains why the health services are full of unreadable publications – leaflets written by doctors for other doctors rather than patients, scientific articles written by French doctors for other French professors rather than American editors, policy documents written for more senior bureaucrats rather than the more junior ones who will have to carry out the plans.

49

But the false feedback loop can be controlled:

- *Make sure that whoever is reading your manuscript knows the audience you are addressing.* This should at least encourage them to make their suggestions with the end-users in mind (*see* **evidence-based writing**).
- *Remember that you are the reader's advocate, and assess all feedback accordingly.* Give in graciously over proposed changes that will not affect the chances of the document being read and acted upon; resist tactfully – and with evidence – those that are likely to turn your audience away (*see* **negotiating changes**).

Feature article   Writing for magazines and newspapers has traditionally been divided into **news stories** and feature articles. Feature articles tend to allow more comment. They also tend to be longer, which is the reason for the most important difference – the structure.

A news story will start with a strong **message**, and then add supporting information in decreasing order of importance (*see* **inverted triangle**). The feature article, being longer, has to have a more sophisticated structure designed to guide the reluctant reader through to the end. There are three elements.

- *Introduction.* The opening is not a gentle statement of what is to come, but the first (and possibly only) opportunity to involve the uncommitted. A common way is to start with a personal story: 'John Smith has always been worried about his appetite. Until now.' After a few paragraphs the writer can raise a question and set up a dynamic: 'So is a diet of carrot juice and boiled rice the best preparation for a marathon run in Antarctica?'.
- *Development.* This is how we get from the introduction to the conclusion: it is the difficult bit. We need to plan a small number of steps, each corresponding with a paragraph, that will develop our argument. Explain each step in the first sentence before going on in the rest of the paragraph to elaborate, illustrate or explain (*see* **yellow marker test**).
- *Conclusion.* At the end of the article the writer will generally leave the reader with a clear conclusion (or **message**), such as: 'The carrot and rice diet is not only good for ice-cold marathons; it also reduces hair loss.'

Features are a broad category. If you are asked to write one, study the publication before you start (*see* **evidence-based writing**). Make sure you understand precisely what the editor wants (*see* **commissioning**).

Follow the usual principles for the **process of writing**. For more information, *see* **journalism booklist**.

Feedback   *See* **balanced feedback; false feedback loop.**

Figures   *See* **illustrations.**

Final sentence   Many people feel that they have to end on a high note. They are right when it comes to **feature articles, review articles, editorials** and **scientific papers**. However, for **memos, letters, news stories, press releases** and **executive summaries**, the message should be shamelessly sold in the first sentence (*see* **inverted triangle structure**). For these types of writing, the final sentence can be the dullest.

Finishing   *See* **getting finished.**

First draft   The defining moment for a piece of writing, when the jumble of ideas in our head has to be put down in some sort of order. We often find it difficult to get through this stage, and have all kinds of strategies for putting it off (*see* **free writing, writer's block**).

First person   This is the grammatical term for using 'I' and 'we' rather than 'you', 'he', 'she', or (if one is royal) 'one'. Many great works of literature have been written in the first person; those writing scientific papers, on the other hand, feel that it is vulgar and detracts from science as an objective pursuit (*see* **voice**). In fact journals are beginning to accept, and in some cases encourage, the first person, particularly in the methods, as in, 'In this study we found ...'. Look in your target journal (*see* **evidence-based writing**).

First sentence   The purpose of this is generally to attract passing trade (*see* **inverted triangle**). Scientific papers are an exception to this rule (*see* **IMRAD; topic sentences**).

First six words test   This is a simple test, based on the assumption that, to read a whole sentence, a whole paragraph or (heavens above!) a whole piece of writing, we have to start by reading the first few words. This test involves reading out loud the first six, and asking the question: 'Could I persuade more people to start reading if I were to use different words?'.

Weak openings would include: 'Considerable debate surrounds the effect of ...' or 'Although many studies have examined aspects ...'. You will find it easy to increase the impact of your first sentence by turning it around, as in: 'The effect of red wine on health has been assimilated in many studies.'

Fish and chip wrappers   One of the great consolations for those who dabble in the imperfect craft of writing (*see* **law of late literals**) is the thought that what is read and digested today will tomorrow be wrapping something that is eaten and digested tomorrow.

Flabby phrases   There are countless words or phrases, such as 'general public', 'at this moment in time', 'a redundancy situation' that we use all the time. That is why it is important to leave time for **rewriting**.

Fog scores   *See* **readability scores**.

Fortune   You are unlikely to make one of these out of your writing, unless you are Jeffrey Archer. You might consider this an unacceptable price to pay (*see* **careers in writing**).

Fraud   *See* **scientific fraud**.

Freelance   A writer who is not on the staff of a publication, but who is paid for contributions. Some doctors like to use this word as an insult, on the grounds that anyone not drawing regular income must be treated with suspicion. Journalists tend to use the term as a compliment, on the grounds that someone can't be that bad if they have got the courage to leave the boring world of office grind and live entirely on their ability to write.

That said, there is no bar to anyone ringing up and saying that they are a freelance journalist. If you happen to be approached by one, ask which journal they are writing for, and whether the article has been commissioned. This should help you make up your mind as to whether to trust them with your opinions, or not.

Free writing   A splendid technique that allows you to write creatively. Go into a room, without any distractions such as reference books or photocopied articles or even the original data, and start to write. You may find it particularly difficult to put down the first sentence, in which case you should put down any old sentence, such as, 'I am sitting here trying to write about ...'.

The trick is to get started so, once started, keep going. When you have finished one sentence, move on at once to writing the next. Resist the pull to look back at what you have just written and start fiddling with it. You should be developing your ideas, and not playing with the punctuation. If you find this impossible, cover up your writing so that you can not look back; if you write straight onto a computer, turn off the screen.

You should be able to write about 30 words a minute in this way, so in 20 minutes you will have drafted 600 or so words. Stop at a set time (use a kitchen timer if you have one). If you haven't finished when your allotted time is up, just sketch out the paragraph headings until the end.

My experience encouraging people to do 10 minutes free writing on a training course is that they find it threatening and difficult for the first two minutes, then become completely absorbed. Often they start to write about things that they did not realize they knew about: in other words they started to unleash their creativity.

People are fairly suspicious of what they have written in this way. But they usually find that their message has come across clearly, and that the structure (as identified by the **yellow marker test**) is unusually well-paced and clear.

There are two caveats. Free writing works well if it is preceded by **planning**; otherwise it is a process of free thinking (*see* **branching**). Second, you will almost certainly need to do further work on your draft. But, now you have coaxed it out of your head and onto a screen or piece of paper, you have something to work with.

Full stops   Also called full points. Harold Evans, the eminent editor of the *Sunday Times* in the 1960s and 1970s, wrote in his book 'The full stop is a great help to sanity'. (*Newsman's English*, Harold Evans, London: Heinemann, 1972, p. 20). Quite.

There is another use for the full stop, and that is when you are using abbreviations. This use seems to be declining and many publications now use the style of 'Mr' or 'eg' (rather than Mr. or e.g.). Be guided by your target publication (*see* **evidence-based writing**).

Fun   If you are not enjoying yourself, how do you expect your readers to?

Getting finished   Perfectionists will keep fiddling with what they have written for ever. The best way of getting out of this loop, and actually finishing, is to set a **deadline**.

Getting started   This is much harder than getting finished. As a general rule, work towards putting words down on paper where you have a chance of controlling and developing them (*see* **process of writing; writer's block**).

Ghost author   This term is used to describe a professional writer who has done most of the work on a piece of writing and who may or may not be given any credit. In the world of scientific journals this is a contentious area, because of the increasing pressure among individuals and organizations to have articles published in the top journals. From an ethical point of view, there doesn't seem to be any problem with this practice, provided that:

- the listed first author has had a major intellectual involvement with the study (*see* **authorship**);
- any company sponsorship is clearly declared (*see* **conflict of interest**), and

- the named authors realize that they have accepted responsibility for the paper (*see* **gift authors**).

Gift author   Someone who has his or her name at the top of an article, but who has not had a major intellectual involvement. This is not considered fair (*see* **authorship; ghost author**).

Gobbledegook   This term, originally from the US and probably inspired by the language of turkeys, is often used to describe language that is overblown, pompous and virtually meaningless, as in: 'At the same time, these contexts of interpretation are themselves ongoing accomplishments, reflexively supplying meaning to actions and objects as those meanings maintain, elaborate or alter the circumstances in which they occur.' The term 'gobbledegook' is usually considered to have the same meaning as **jargon**. However, I think a useful distinction can be made, which is that jargon is essentially technical language, used inappropriately. Gobbledegook is just old-fashioned rubbish.

Good writing   *See* **effective writing**.

Grammar   Grammar is simply the set of rules needed to ensure that, when one person says or writes something in a particular language, others sharing that language will understand. Most of us are pretty good at it. We may not be able to parse, or decline, or identify the parts of speech, but we do manage to use the rules to put our messages across.

Yet most of us think that we are pretty bad at it, and some of our colleagues waste no time in trying to convince us of this. These people scan the writing of others like hawks, swooping on fairly unimportant deviations (like **split infinitives**) and using them to demotivate the writer and devalue the writing.

Fortunately there are several strategies you can adopt to produce well-grammared sentences (a bad example of **verbing** – *see* **verbs**). If you are really keen, buy a book – not one of those thick tomes with acres of small print on the finer points, but a short book, for children or foreigners or journalists, that gives you the main rules. Alternatively, use the grammar checker on your computer. These are getting much better than they used to be, and you don't even have to have studied grammar at school to work out what you need to put it right. Finally, if you are part of that group of people who went to school when it was fashionable not to teach grammar, you should make sure you get help. Find someone who will love going through what you have written, and 'making it grammatical'.

Getting help, from whatever source, isn't cheating: it's sensible **project management**.

BOOKLIST: grammar and usage

- *English for journalists* (2nd edition), by Wynford Hicks, London: Routledge, 1998. Most books on grammar consist of long and complicated lists and are completely indigestible. This book is blessedly short, with the author whizzing through the basic rules of grammar in 12 pages. It is aimed at journalists but useful to a much wider audience.

- *Fowler's modern English usage* (3rd edition), edited by RW Burchfield, Oxford: Oxford University Press, 1996. The cover proclaims that this is 'the acknowledged authority on English usage'. Useful to dip into, but don't try reading it in one go.

- *The good English guide*, by Godfrey Howard, London: Macmillan, 1993. Similar to Fowler's. For reasons that I find it hard to identify (it may simply be a matter of typeface), it seems less stuffy.

- *The complete plain words* (3rd edition), by Sir Ernest Gowers, revised by Sidney Greenbaum and Janet Whitcut, London: HMSO, 1986. Originally written to encourage civil servants to write in plain English, this book gives plenty of good advice on writing clear English. I recommend buying a departmental copy that can be used to settle matters in dispute.

- *Troublesome words*, by Bill Bryson, London: Penguin (revised) 1999. A highly readable reference work showing the idiosyncrasies of the English language. An early voyage by a subsequently famous travel writer.

Grant applications

Careers depend on persuading organizations with funds to give support, so these are extremely important pieces of writing. There is no magic formula, and grant applications should be approached in the same way as any other pieces of writing (*see* **process of writing**). I have six particular points to make.

- *Find the right organization to approach.* Many directories will give you information, and your colleagues should also be able to help you. One of the best ways is to identify the key papers in your field (defined as tightly as possible) and try to find out where the funding came from. Target these organizations: a fundamental law of selling states that it is easier to make a sale from someone who has already bought (and seen the benefits of) a similar product.

- *Invest time in researching the market.* You cannot research too thoroughly what the organization wants. Ask for, and read carefully, any literature that they produce, in particular guidelines for those submitting proposals. Try to find out what they have given money to, and if possible get hold of those proposals in order to analyse the **structure** and **style**. This is as important as researching the topic you wish to investigate.

- *Work out carefully the message you would like to give if your research is successful.* Grant-giving organizations get no points for giving out money; they do get points for funding work that can be seen to have moved forward our knowledge of science, or (particularly if patient groups are involved) have had a demonstrable clinical effect. Work backwards: what **headlines** would you hope your research to attract (provided all goes well)? Use these thoughts to inform your **message,** and make sure that your message is clearly given when you write your application.

- *Make time for your submission.* This is extremely important, so don't treat it as something to be bolted on to your life at the end of the working day. Put aside time so that you can do this properly (*see* **time management**).

- *If your application is unsuccessful, learn from it.* Many organizations will give you **feedback**. Study it carefully. Was the work flawed scientifically, in which case can you remedy it? Was it sent to the wrong organization, in which case how do you find out the right one? Did it fail to inspire the panel, in which case was it because you failed to make clear the amazing implications – or was it a run-of-the-mill idea that will not advance anything very much and therefore will prove difficult to fund?

- *Make the most of a successful application.* Don't be bashful: everyone loves a success (well, up to a point) and you should unashamedly use yours to advance your own interests. Throw a party, and invite all those whom you wish to impress.

Gravitas   The ability to make the commonplace sound original and impressive. Good for glittering careers, but hardly reader-friendly (*see* **putting on the posh overcoat**).

Great writers   These are born and not made. This book deals with writing as a craft not an art, so 'greatness' is beyond its scope. Good enough will do (*see* **effective writing**).

Green ink brigade   There is a prejudice among many editors that those who write in green ink are mad. This is not evidence based. Until someone does the definitive study, however, if you write a letter to an editor, hide your ink preference by using a word processor.

Gut reaction   The main way in which editors choose articles for their journal – a feeling that it is somehow 'more right' for their readers than the alternatives. This is what they get paid for. Although the system is not scientific, it is as good as any other system of selection – perhaps better.

Hanging participles   *See* **dangling modifiers**.

Hard copy   Text that appears on paper rather than being electronically stored and presented. Those of us of a certain age remain sentimentally attached to it.

Headlines   There is a useful distinction to make between titles and headlines. Titles (as appearing on the top of scientific papers) are labels that identify what the writing covers, but (with the exception of **declarative titles**) they do not give away, or try to sell, the **message**. They are an invitation to those who are interested to read further.

Headlines play a more aggressive role: their task is to attract more than just committed readers and therefore their function is to *sell* the message so that casual readers will want to find out more. They are not summary, but advertising, 'Too much salt kills baby fed cheap diet' and 'SHAME OF SMOKER MUMS' may appear garish to those brought up on science journals, and the messages may not be to everyone's taste. But they are clearly stated, and there's a good case for arguing that this is better than no credible message at all (*see* **Pravda effect**).

The job of **subeditors** on newspapers and magazines is to write these headlines. They often have to do this to tight **deadlines,** and on copy where the message is not always clear. They also have to write to very tight design specifications – such as (in the first story above) four lines of no more than 10 characters each.

These design considerations mean that, when you submit an article, the title you choose is unlikely to make it through to publication. Yet it will be on the headline that your peers will focus their critical powers (*see* **false feedback loop**). Don't be put off: ask them if they read the story underneath. If they say 'yes', then count it as a victory for you and your subeditor.

Heartsink writer   Some writers always know better than their editors, never accept no for an answer, keep arguing and generally behave like the worst kind of patient. Avoid such behaviour (*see* **dealing with editors**).

Holiday writing   *See* **travel writing**.

Homophones   When it comes to words, there are many **confusing pairs**; homophones are those that sound the same, such as:
- *born* and *borne*: (1) arriving in this world, and (2) carried,
- *complementary* and *complimentary*: (1) something that adds, and (2) something that is free or giving praise,
- *discreet* and *discrete*: (1) not likely to gossip, and (2) each separate piece,
- *principal* and *principle*: (1) main (person), and (2) a rule,
- *stationary* and *stationery*: (1) at a standstill, and (2) envelopes and writing paper.

House style   *See* **Instructions to Authors; style guide.**

However   Some people get really worked up as to whether 'however' is allowed to go at the front of a sentence or not. Others feel it's not worth wasting time on. Which sentence brings us to another question: should we be ending sentences with prepositions? Who cares (*see* **English teachers**)?

Humiliation   Some see this as an essential part of commenting on what another person has written (*see* **balanced feedback; politics of writing**).

Hyphens   These give rise to two main problems:
- *whether to put them in at all*. Currently it is fashionable to leave them out. This leads to phrases such as 'a primary health care led NHS' that are virtually impossible to understand at first reading. As a general guide, put them in to help the reader group words correctly, or to avoid ambiguity (last-minute changes or last minute changes?).
- *layout*. When narrow columns are being used, many of the words become split over two lines, and therefore hyphenated. This can turn the right-hand margin into a succession of small horizontal lines. In the old days, when type was set by hand, typesetters could take time and care to avoid this by subtle manipulation of letters and spaces. Now the computers seem to be in control: there seems to be little we can do to change this. Try to ignore it.

Icarus fallacy   In Greek mythology, Icarus was the one who soared nearer and nearer to the sun. Unfortunately, while the notion of building wings was ingenious and the construction of them skilful, the theory was based on a major miscalculation: his wings were made of feathers and wax, and when he flew near to the sun the wax melted and he fell back to earth.

This triumph of optimism over advance planning seems appropriate to describe the assumption that a scientific paper, once launched, can soar higher and higher towards excellence. Thus an article which started out fit for the *Northumberland Digest of Dull Medicine* will eventually, with 'high quality' (i.e. painstaking and painful) advice from colleagues and professors, have the editors of the *New England Journal* and *The Lancet* fighting over it.

This of course is just not true. It is almost always possible to work out how 'good' a paper will be (i.e. which journal is likely to publish it) before you start to write the first draft (*see* **brief setting**). If the basics are not there before you write (i.e. the idea is not original enough, or the numbers too small) it is unlikely to change during the **process of writing**.

Ideas   The problem is usually having too many of them, rather than not having any at all (*see* **rumination**).

Illness   Many people find it helpful to write about the illness of themselves or of a loved one. As with **travel writing**, the supply greatly exceeds the demand. Your chances of getting an article of this kind published increase considerably if you can draw out of the particular case some general message. But don't let this deter you: on these occasions you should be writing for yourself, and regarding publication as an unlikely bonus. *See also* **case notes**.

Illustrations   When writing for scientific papers, you will be expected to provide these, when appropriate. Take guidance from the **Instructions to Authors** and from the **Vancouver group** guidelines. If you are using pictures of patients, make sure that you have their written consent.

When writing for magazines and newspapers, you will not normally be expected to provide photographs and illustrations: the editorial staff will organize these. The exception is if you have taken photographs, for instance on an expedition to the North Pole, that cannot be replicated.

A useful principle when submitting illustrations, particularly valuable ones, is that anything that can be lost will be lost. Keep the original and send a copy.

Impact factor   Eugene Garfield hit on the idea of measuring a journal's worth by working out how often the papers it publishes are cited by other journals. This is now a huge enterprise, undertaken by the Institute for Scientific Information in its annual *Journal Citation Reports*. But despite the elegance of the idea, impact factors have had a baleful influence on medical writing.

As a measure of **quality**, of course, the index is suspect because it modifies the human behaviour it tries to measure. Most of those involved with science publishing agree that the system favours US journals, and that individual editors from all over the world directly and indirectly encourage authors to cite from their own journal. The whole thing becomes self-fulfilling as those with high scores attract the best pieces, and those with a lower index start to struggle.

As for writers, impact factors have encouraged them to choose publications on the basis of the points they are likely to get rather than because of the audience they would like to reach. It encourages them – and their co-authors – to hold out for a high impact journal, even though any rational view would tell them that the work in hand is simply not appropriate (*see* **Icarus fallacy**). Some departments now send their article routinely to the higher impact journals, rationalizing it by saying that at least they will get a high quality review. But it doesn't seem a sensible use of anybody's time and money.

IMRAD structure   The model was originally proposed by the British scientist Bradford Hill, and the idea was to help writers by using a simple four-part structure. Each section answers a simple question.

- *Introduction – or why did we start?* The typical introduction consists of two or three paragraphs. Despite what many people think, the **first sentence** is generally dull and can be divided into three types: (1) the Seminar Approach ('Left-handedness is a condition affecting 10% of the population ...'); (2) the Alarmist ('Hundreds of left-handed people commit suicide each year claiming that they cannot get their scientific papers published, and the figure is rising'), and (3) Much Discussion Recently ('There has been much discussion recently about the impact of being-left-handed on the task of writing scientific papers'). The most important sentence in the Introduction, therefore, is not the first one but the last, which typically describes what the authors did: 'In this study we conducted a postal survey of 2 million doctors to see if there was a link between authorship and left-handedness.'

- *Methods – or what did we do?* This section usually consists of about six to seven paragraphs, though journals concentrating on pure research may often take longer. This section is straightforward and describes exactly what you did. The descriptions should be full enough to allow someone else to replicate what you did. Avoid woolly phrases like 'within five minutes of Birmingham ...'. If necessary divide this section into subsections.
- *Results – or what did you find?* This section tends to consist of six to seven paragraphs. It will almost certainly refer you to **figures** and **tables**. You need to comment on these, and draw attention to the main trends.
- *Discussion – or what does it all mean?* The first sentence plays a key role and describes the main findings: 'In this study we found clear evidence that those who write with their left hand are far less likely to have scientific papers published.' It then moves on to put these conclusions in context, with each paragraph dealing with a different point (such as the reasons for the link and how this relates to existing theories; the implications of this finding to medical science and society; the future direction of work; the day-to-day implications for clinical work, etc). Sometimes there may be as many as seven to eight paragraphs, each dealing with a particular aspect. The **final sentence** should be conclusive, and in about 50% of articles it does give a clear conclusion or message: 'Left-handed people should be given extra assistance if we are to expect them to write as many papers as other people.' About one quarter are what I have called 'perhaps possibly' endings: 'Left-handedness could possibly, under certain conditions, be one of several influences affecting the publication of scientific papers' (*Winning the publications game – see* **scientific papers booklist**). A final quarter seem to have no real conclusion other than they should carry on with their work (*see* '**more research is indicated**').

However, while IMRAD is a useful structure for authors to follow, it is not reader-friendly. The main message is at the end (if at all) which is not a logical place to put it. (The abstract doesn't help, because it follows the same structure). However, the last two or three generations of scientists have become used to it, and therefore if you want to communicate with them then you must conform to that structure. Under no circumstances, however, should you use this structure for anything other than original scientific papers, and perhaps some papers for other professionals who are somehow expecting that you write this way. Wherever possible prefer the **inverted triangle**.

Individuality   Some feel that their writing should reflect their own personality. The trouble is that they end up writing to please themselves, not the reader (*see* **false feedback loop**).

Infinitives, split   *See* **split infinitives.**

Instructions to Authors   Most academic journals publish a wide range of specific rules on what contributions they seek and how they wish to have them presented (*see* **style guide**). These are drawn together, under the heading of 'Instructions to Authors', and published in each edition of the journal or at regular and well-publicized intervals. Most of them go into considerable detail, with instructions on the size of paper, how to lay out the first page, copyright and reprints, and the number and style of references.

They also give useful insights into the culture of a journal. For instance, the instructions in the *International Journal of Epidemiology* state that the journal 'publishes original work, reviews and letters to the Editor in the fields of research and teaching in epidemiology'. The *European Journal of Epidemiology*, on the other hand, 'serves as a forum on the epidemiology of communicable and non-communicable diseases and their control'. Such differences, although subtle, can give useful information to those planning where they should target their paper.

From the writer's point of view, it is vital that you obey these instructions to the letter. This should not be a problem if you make sure that you do not write a paper without first deciding where you wish it to be published (*see* **brief setting**); indeed the instructions should make things clearer and easier. One warning, however: when it comes to working out the precise market requirements of a journal, the Instructions to Authors are only one part of the picture. There are many aspects of a paper, such as the way in which the title is written, or the favoured style, that can be discovered only by careful analysis of the papers published in your target journal (*see* **evidence-based writing**).

Integrity   *See* **editorial integrity; scientific fraud.**

International Committee of Medical Journal Editors
See **Vancouver Group.**

Internet   *See* **World Wide Web**.

Interviewing   The ability to carry out a good interview gives writers a valuable tool. It enables them to gather information quickly from those who have expertise in a given area, and in a language that, because it is informal and spoken, is more likely to pass the **pub test** and be accessible to the target readers.

The quality of an interview, however, depends on how well you have chosen the person to be interviewed. The best way is to ask other people. Don't go to the experts only; you need people who can communicate in clear English. Watch for biases and hidden agendas – and if possible balance one expert with another.

Once you have found your interviewee, the following step-by-step plan should be helpful:

- *Be absolutely clear before you start what you want to achieve.* There are, broadly speaking, three reasons for an interview: (1) to get facts and information; (2) to add opinion or description to facts that you already have, and (3) to provide information for a profile of the interviewee. For each of these, you will need a different set of questions.

- *Prepare the interview carefully, in a way that will not restrict you later.* Use a technique such as **branching** to work out the information you need, and use this to construct a checklist of questions. Group these questions into three or four broad areas and either memorize this summary or write it down on a piece of paper. Check your equipment: most writers have etched on their memories the disastrous times when they discovered that their tape recorder had broken, or had to borrow a pen or some pieces of paper from the interviewee.

- *Give a good impression from the start.* Interviews are not the time to make a fashion statement: the more acceptable you appear to the interviewee, the more likely you will be to get good quality information. Make your interviewee feel comfortable. Start with some small talk and easy questions. This is the time to set any ground rules (*see* **off the record**; **non-attributable information**). These should be negotiated before you start rather than when the questions start getting difficult.

- *Throughout the interview remain firmly in control.* Follow your agenda, not that of the interviewee. But don't get tied into a long list of questions: using a summary rather than the full list will help you to be more flexible. Keep the interviewee on track, though sometimes desperate measures may be needed, such as knocking over a glass of water. Using a tape recorder will free you to concentrate on the business in hand – though keep some written notes as well, just in case there is a systems failure.

- *Close the interview in a positive way.* Make a checklist of important points, such as 'Anything else to add?', 'Should I talk to anyone else?' and 'How can I contact you within the next 24 hours?'. Interviewees will often ask to see a copy of what you have written before it is published. The danger with this is that they will try to get rid of their bright, clear quotes and try to put back their posh overcoat (*see* **putting on the posh overcoat**). On the other hand, passing your copy to them will probably pick up one or two errors of fact. Use your discretion: a sensible compromise is to read what you have written over the phone. In that way they can pick up errors but will have no time to fiddle with the style.
- *Review what you have been told as soon as possible after the interview.* Wherever possible go through the information as soon as the interview is over. When you come to write, you should be in a position to take out of it, from memory, what you need. Avoid where possible writing up transcripts: this takes up huge amounts of time.

If you come out of your interview feeling humiliated, don't worry. The test of a good interviewer is not what the interviewee thinks, but the quality of the information elicited, or the liveliness of the **quotes**.

Introductions   Many people believe that the role of the first part of a piece of writing is to introduce the reader to what you are going to say so that the reader can decide whether or not to become involved. This probably stems from school essays and has a slightly old-fashioned feel to it. For most types of writing (though see **IMRAD** above for an important exception) use the first sentence far more aggressively, as a hook to get the reader's interest. If readers don't become involved in the first sentence, they almost certainly won't become involved in the second (*see* **intro; inverted triangle**).

Intro   This is the term used by journalists to describe the **first sentence** of a **news story**. It is constructed using the **inverted triangle** model.

Inverted triangle   This is the structure, also called the news pyramid, taught to generations of journalism students. It is based on the assumption that your best chance of being read is to put your finest information into the first sentence. Once you have done that, you can put in all the qualifying information, in order of importance.

The occasional (or perhaps more than occasional, depending on the papers you buy) lapses into extremity should not distract from the fact that this is a sensible approach, and we should adopt it for many types of writing up to about 400 words – particularly **letters, e-mails** and **executive summaries** (*see* **marketing**).

Jargon   This is one of those things that – like smoking, obesity and other people's fast cars – we are all against. But it is not a clear concept. It is derived from a French word that described the twittering of birds, and in the mid-19th century the famous war correspondent Russell could use the phrase 'the jargon of the campfires' in his description of the scene on the night before battle.

Much of what we call jargon today is actually a technical language that has a precise meaning for fellow professionals, but is meaningless to outsiders. Doctors talk of ESRs and perinatal mortalities. Sociologists talk of normative structures and *anomie*. Trainers talk of talking walls and problem-based learning. All have meanings within their group and are useful because they can describe complex notions and ideas in a simple way. The difficulty comes when these terms are used inappropriately to the wrong audiences.

A slightly different type of writing, also called jargon by some people, is the flabby and pompous: 'Further to my previous correspondence, in respect of your dissatisfaction with your recent holiday in our facility, I can confirm that I have investigated this matter fully and comprehensively and will now endeavour to clarify the points you raised.' This is not a technical language, but a succession of empty phrases, and I think are better described as **gobbledegook**.

Jargon (as opposed to gobbledegook) has proliferated because of the increasing tendency to write one document for a number of different audiences (*see* **effective writing**), or even for the wrong audience (*see* **false feedback loop**). The answer is not to get rid of all these uncommon words completely, but to make sure that we use the right language for our audience. If we do this, the jargon problem will go away.

Jokes   It is difficult to make these work in the unforgiving black and white of the printed word. If you want to risk one, tell it economically and quickly. Test it on someone else before launching it to the general readership – and believe them if they say that it's not funny.

Journalese   Doctors often use this word as a general term of abuse for vulgar and sensational writing. Journalists use it to describe words that are so over-used that they have become **clichés** – from 'official sources revealed yesterday' to 'top docs probe mercy dash blaze horror' (*see* **journalism**).

Journalism   At its worst the hounder of innocent princesses and enemy of sensible government. At its best the exposer of unprincipled villains and deposers of evil regimes. Whether you love it or loathe it, the practice of journalism provides some useful lessons for those wishing to learn how to communicate effectively (*see* **tabloids**). It also provides major opportunities for putting out important public health messages (*see* **press releases**).

BOOKLIST: journalism

- *The fight for public health*, by Simon Chapman and Deborah Lupton, London: BMJ Books, 1994. A must for doctors who wish to influence public health. Written by two experienced campaigners it shows how the mass media, if understood and used properly, can put across immensely powerful public health messages.
- *Medical journalism; the writer's guide*, by Tim Albert, Abingdon: Radcliffe Medical Press, 1992. This book tries to explain how doctors can learn to write for magazines and newsletters rather than journals.
- *Communicating science: a handbook*, by Michael Shortland and Jane Gregory, London: Longman, 1991. An excellent and provocative book intended to cajole scientists into communicating properly, whether by writing, speaking or 'meeting the media'.

- *Writing feature articles*, by Brendan Hennessy, Oxford: Heinemann, 1989. Professional exposition of how to write feature articles for newspapers and magazines.
- *Health writer's handbook*, by Barbara Gastel, Iowa: Iowa State University Press, 1998. Dr Gastel runs a master's degree programme in science and technology journalism and this is a useful account of what is happening in the United States.

Journals   All over the world thousands of journals are published each year, most run by commercial organizations, but some in partnership with professional associations. They contain a blend of material, such as **editorials, review articles, letters, obituaries** and **news,** but what distinguishes them from **magazines** is that they include **scientific papers** sent out for **peer review.**

Originally set up to inform 'artisan countrymen and merchants' of the developments of science, they later narrowed their focus to smaller and smaller groups of colleagues. More recently, through the development of peer review, they have played a key role in validating science (and scientists). In the last few years **electronic publishing** has challenged a number of assumptions, such as the fact that space to publish is limited and that reviewing can be done only before publication.

We are in for some dramatic changes. One of the most likely scenarios seems to be the increasing use of electronic publishing to validate science, and (with luck) the return of journals to their original purpose of communicating exciting advances of knowledge. Whatever happens, the need to understand **effective writing** will not go away.

BOOKLIST: journals

- *Journal publishing* by Gillian Page, Robert Campbell and Jack Meadows, Cambridge: Cambridge University Press, 1997. The standard work.
- *Peer review in health sciences*, edited by Fiona Godlee and Tom Jefferson: London: BMJ Books, 1999. Unlikely to help anyone with their writing problems, but will delight the fans of peer review.
- *The future of medical journals*, edited by Stephen Lock, London: BMJ Books, 1991. Published to mark the retirement of Stephen Lock as editor of the BMJ, this book has a range of provocative and entertaining articles on all aspects of medical

69

journals. It is particularly interesting to look back at how Richard Smith, the current editor, predicted the development of journals.

Journalology　The word used to describe the study of matters of interest to editors of learned journals. These include **authorship, reviewing,** and **scientific fraud**. Readability, alas, rarely figures highly.

KISS　Keep It Short and Simple. And there's no better guide than this if you want to cultivate an effective writing style.

Key words　These are the half dozen or so words that you need to include with an article in order to aid electronic retrieval. The **Vancouver Group** define them as 'key words or short phrases that will assist indexers in cross indexing the article and may be published with the abstract. Terms from the medical subject headlines (MeSH) list of *Index Medicus* should be used.'

They are important. If you don't have the right key words, then all the work you have done will float out on the electronic highway, unread and adding nothing to the sum of human knowledge.

Kill fee　If a commissioned article is returned unused authors will sometimes receive a kill fee to compensate them for the time spent (*see* **commissioning**).

Latin education　Not a good preparation for those who want to be able to write effective contemporary English. It encourages a nostalgic loyalty towards Latin and Greek words rather than the Anglo-Saxon – 'commence' rather than 'start', 'participate' rather than 'take part'. It also encourages the peculiarly ornate constructions favoured by Latin textbooks: 'Having attacked Labienus with arrows, Cotta rolled bundles into the ditch' (*see* **dangling modifier**). Finally, Latin is no longer a developing language and therefore can encourage the delusion that language has immutable rules (*see* **pub test**).

Latin plurals   Insisting on these has become an affectation. But those who insist that 'data' are plural are unlikely to say 'We should renew our insurance premia' or 'Please turn to agendum number one.' Be guided by common usage and ignore the snobs.

Law of late literals   At least one mistake in every piece of writing will be discovered once it is too late to do anything about it. The only consolation is to think of all the things you did get right (*see* **proofreading; spelling**).

Lawyers   It is usually best to avoid their interventions (*see* **copyright; libel**) – but beware falling into the trap of **defensive writing**.

Lay person   A put-down by those in one group to describe members of another. The difference is usually made to seem greater than it is by the use of jargon.

Layout   How we lay out what we write on a page has an enormous influence on how it will be received, and you can ruin much hard work by thoughtless presentation. Here are some principles.
- *Follow the style of your organization.* Many people like to feel that they need to exercise their individuality and therefore must ignore any style laid down by the organization they work for. Resist this temptation, partly because it is in both your interests and those of your organization to keep a consistent image. Those who have decided on your corporate image will usually have had training in design and therefore will probably have a better idea of what works (not that you will believe them).

- *Use white space carefully.* White space should be used to frame words, not to interrupt them. Avoid white space between paragraphs. Make sure the margins round the outside of the page are wide enough to give an air of organization. And keep to them: don't change the margins in order to accommodate extra words; get rid of some words.
- *Choose one main typeface and stick to it.* Research on readability is clear: it doesn't matter which of the main **typefaces** you use, as long as you use it large enough (12 point if you are using the width of an A4 sheet) and don't play around (*see* **polyfontophilia**). You may wish to use a second typeface for headings and other devices, but don't overdo it. Look at publications you enjoy reading, and those you should read and don't, and see what design differences there are.
- *Make the most of modern technology.* Word processing packages can do all kinds of wonderful things and, provided you don't get carried away, can make things much easier for the target reader. There are few remaining excuses for the illegible scribbled note.
- *Avoid crossings out.* In the old days, if you made a mistake, you had to get out a bottle of correcting fluid or simply tear out the sheet and start again. Now all you have to do is make a change and run off another copy. So there should be no excuse for submitting copy with handwritten amendments: it looks messy, and sends a strong message that the writing and thinking will be messy, too.

Leaf shuffling

Some people write as if they were building a tree. But instead of starting with the trunk and then adding the branches, they get a whole pile of leaves (such as data or references) and start moving them around. And around. And around. This is an interesting form of **writer's block**, particularly since those who suffer from this affliction can plead that they are meticulous researchers. It rarely advances the **writing process**.

Leaving things out

The real problem in writing is leaving things out, not putting them in (*see* **leaf shuffling**).

Length

Depends on what the reader can take (or what your editor thinks the reader can take), and not what you want to give (*see* **brief setting**).

Letters   We all write these. Some, like the complaint about the poor service on the flight, are relatively easy; others (like answering the complaint) are less so. The principles are generally the same as for other formats (*see* process **of writing**), but the following specific points should help.

- *Be clear about what you are trying to achieve.* Is the purpose of the letter to answer a complaint, for instance, in which case you can consider it a success if you hear no more about it? Or is it to invite someone to do something, in which case your success can be measured by whether they do it (*see* **brief setting**)?
- *Be clear about the real audience.* In a few cases, the person to whom you are ostensibly writing the letter will not be your real audience. It could be a lawyer, or your superior. Being clear about this before you start will help you to avoid failing to please either.
- *Use the right tone.* Once you have decided on your audience, write as if you were speaking directly to him or her. This should not be seen as an opportunity to impress (*see* **putting on the posh overcoat**).
- *Cough if you have to.* It is considered polite in some English letter writing circles to preface your remarks with a polite cough: 'Thank you for your letter', 'It was good to see you', or 'I am writing to ...'. This is fine, but don't overdo it.
- *Give your message as soon as you can.* Immediately after your cough, tell the reader what is going to be in it for him or her: ' I am delighted to say that your complaint has been upheld', or 'I am writing to you with an invitation to invest £1 million in my institute so that we can finally find the cure for the common cold.'
- *Use the language of your reader.* Unless you deliberately want to scare off the recipient of your letter (*see* **political writing**), use the words and constructions that you think he or she will be comfortable with. Don't worry about being **patronizing**; do worry about being **pompous**.
- *Exceed one page at your peril.* Most people say that they like one side of paper only, so do what they ask. Brevity of course always takes a little longer, but you will normally find it worth the effort.
- *Take care with presentation.* Follow your **house style**, and use a reader-friendly **layout**. Remember that it is the design, not the words, that will give the first impression. Don't spoil it by, for instance, cramped margins and tiny type. Whenever possible, sign the letter yourself.
- *Leave it overnight if it is a sensitive matter.* Important letters are worth taking time and trouble over. Leave it for a while,

73

preferably overnight. This applies particularly to letters written in anger: by the next day a less confrontational alternative will usually have suggested itself.

- *Put it in the right envelope.* Stupid things happen, like the welcoming letter that gets posted to the rejected candidate, or the letter with the post-it note still attached, saying, 'This man is a little odd: placate him.' Be careful.

See also **covering letter; resignation letter.**

Letters to the Editor   These are usually fairly short pieces of writing (two to three paragraphs) submitted for publication. They are different from the **covering letter** accompanying articles.

Many people look down on them, which is a shame because they are difficult to do well, and are often more widely read than longer pieces. They give people the chance to write for publication, and, if accepted, to see how their work is used. They also bring the writer to the attention of the publication's editorial staff, which may lead to an article being commissioned in the future.

Look carefully at the letters in the target publication, and work out how long (or how short) it should be. Work out what you want to achieve, and what message you want to give. You will have few words to play with for this so weigh up carefully what you need to say. Go for the big picture: avoid the carping letter full of little gripes. And if you can, end on a note of humour. But be careful (*see* **jokes**).

Libel   This is **defamation** in written form.

Lies   *See* **scientific fraud.**

Light touch   A gift from the gods and relatively rare. Those who write in this way are often surprised that they can do it, while those who can't will never believe they can't do it. Generally it cannot be taught – but this isn't the same as saying that those who have it don't need to work at it (*see* **rewriting**).

Lists   Many people like to make lists before they start to write. They are making some attempt at planning, which is good. But lists can be limiting: they are one-dimensional and tend to establish links between thoughts and ideas that can be difficult to alter. Some teachers on effective writing techniques now recommend more flexible ways of planning (*see* **branching**).

Literature (1)   The term used to describe a piece of writing that is still read and valued, sometimes centuries after it first appeared, because of some enduring qualities that are often hard to define. It has usually been written because the writer has some kind of impulse to write. It differs from the kind of writing dealt with in this book, where the purpose is not to please the writer (or satisfy his or her demons) but to put a message across to a target audience (*see* **effective writing**).

Literature (2)   A word also used to describe what appears in scientific journals (as in: 'a study of the literature reveals ...'). Since the quality of writing in journals is usually extremely poor (*see* **style**), this is a clever piece of marketing on behalf of the academic community.

Long sentences   Difficult to do well. Those who think they can do them well are usually mistaken.

Long words   Favour shorter ones (*see* **putting on the posh overcoat**).

Macro-editing   This refers to the under-used technique of asking one or two major questions when you are considering a piece of writing in draft, rather than throwing at it all kinds of detailed but minor difficulties (*see* **micro-editing; balanced feedback**).

Magazines   A decade or so ago it used to be easy to distinguish between a magazine and a newspaper – generally the magazine had a picture on the cover, more illustrations inside, greater use of colour and fewer topical news stories. Now the differences are becoming blurred.

Traditionally magazines have been divided into two groups:

- The business press comprises publications sent to specific groups, (such as doctors, lawyers, elevator manufacturers) often without charge.
- The 'consumer' press comprises publications sold over the counter and dealing with all kinds of leisure activities, from crosswords to racing pigeons, from home makeovers to genealogy, and from health to horoscopes. More and more of them have slots for health-related issues.

The basic principle of writing for a magazine is similar to that used for writing for a scientific journal: identify your **market**, create your product, and sell it. The best place to start is those magazines to which you subscribe because presumably you will share the interests and language of the readers. Look for the places where the editor encourages contributions, such as the letters page, special slots such as 'Soapbox' or 'Open Door', or **competitions**. Use the **process of writing** as outlined elsewhere in this book. But bear in mind the following points.

- *There is no peer review system.* A good editor will often seek a second opinion (or third or fourth), but will do so informally. This clarifies your task: you have to please the editor, and not go through a panel of unknown (and therefore unpredictable) reviewers. If you are rejected, however, you will not receive reviewers' comments explaining why.
- *There will rarely be Instructions to Authors.* Most magazines depend on professional contributors, and therefore forgo the practice, common in scientific publications, of printing detailed instructions. You will have to work out for yourself what gets published, and why (*see* **evidence-based writing; marketing**).
- **Readers are considered much more important than authors.** Magazines have to compete with each other for relatively scarce readers – and therefore they go to considerable lengths to ensure that articles are presented in the way they think their readers will like. This means time and effort spent on **subediting**. As a contributor you may disagree with some of these changes, but the subeditors, not you, are the experts in what their readers will be expected to read. If you feel that the subediting has altered your

meaning, there are two possibilities: the subeditor is incompetent (but why has he or she not been fired already?) or you, the author, has failed to be clear enough in the first place. If you cannot live with the changes, seek other outlets for your creativity.

- *Few magazines will send you a proof in advance of publication.* This is very time-consuming and causes many delays and hours of aggravation. Few magazine editors feel that these disadvantages are outweighed by the advantage of spotting one or two errors, usually minor ones.

- *Many magazines will pay for contributions.* The larger magazines (in terms of circulation) will almost certainly pay for publication. Rates will range from about £60 for a small contribution to a small publication to £200 or more for a major national magazine. Most publications have standard amounts, so it is sensible to inquire before you write what you will be paid.

Managing upwards   Unless they also own the publication, editors are employed by an individual or an organization (*see* **bosses**). It is therefore an important part of their role to make sure that they can count on their support. The following techniques are useful.

- *Invest time in getting to know those who could fire you.* This seems fairly self-evident, but the recent history of journals is littered with the firings of editors who had failed to get on with those who had power over them.

- *Hold regular meetings.* These sessions could be formal or informal. They are important because it can give both parties warning if conflict seems to be brewing.

- *Don't provide unpleasant surprises.* If you want to do something controversial, consider informing them in advance, though preferably when it is just too late for them to stop you.

- *Share your successes.* The people we are talking about are not in their posts because of philanthropy; they are there so that they can feel good and successful. When things go right, as they surely must, make sure that they share in the warm afterglow.

- *Have fun.* Build up a culture where, at least once a year, people come together in a relaxing situation. These do not have to be artificial situations like go-karting or rock climbing, but perhaps a reception for contributors, allied with a light-hearted awards ceremony.

Marketing   The kind of writing we are talking about in this book is really marketing – of a piece of information we want to put across, or a request for help of some kind, or simply some advertising for ourselves and our abilities. This has important implications for the writer – in particular it stresses the importance of defining our customer at an early stage (*see* **setting the brief**).

This approach is reassuring when it comes to writing scientific papers. We no longer have to think in terms of passing some quality mark (*see* **Icarus fallacy**), but instead can view what we write simply as a product that has to be sold. The editor becomes a customer, not a judge. This means that we can do market research on what he or she seems to like, by running a literature search on the topic in that journal, or by examining the way articles are presented (*see* **evidence-based writing**), and by studying the **Instructions to Authors**.

Medical newspapers   Doctors are particularly well served by professional newspapers (some would say too well served) mainly because of the advertising support from pharmaceutical companies. I suspect that these newspapers are more influential than many would like to believe (*see* **Pulse phenomenon**).

They also provide excellent opportunities for doctors who want to write. Most parts of these papers (such as the news sections, editorials) are written by the paper's own professional staff, but there are other areas where they positively welcome **feature articles** written by readers. Writing for these papers is an excellent way of learning the crafts of writing and of dealing successfully with editors.

Memos   The person-to-person memo has largely been super-seded by **e-mail**. This still leaves the 'public' memorandum, which comes down from on high, sits at the corner of a notice board until the ends start to curl, and is meant to change group behaviour. As with all other types of writing, make sure you are clear before you start what you are trying to achieve. Perhaps a quiet word, or a good party, will do the trick instead? If you do decide to go ahead, make sure your message is clearly stated in the first sentence (*see* **inverted triangle**).

Message   A fundamental principle that runs throughout this book is that, if you want your readers to emerge with a message and act on what you have written, then the sensible thing to do is to define that message carefully before you start (*see* **brief setting**).

Methodologists   They currently enjoy considerable influence with the editors of medical journals. While no one could sensibly condemn the view that we should make sure that our researches have been conducted properly, there is a danger that dotting every methodological 'i' and crossing every methodological 't' can make us lose sight of the fact that writing is of value only if others can read and understand it. This may explain why there are thousands (millions, even) of papers that, though methodologically sound, are largely ignored (*see* **leaf shuffling**).

Micro-editing   This is the more common approach to giving comments on what others have written. Unlike **macro-editing**, it involves focusing on details rather than important issues. It is over-used (*see* **balanced feedback**).

Mindmapping   The theory and practice of a type of brain-storming devised by Tony Buzan. *See* **brainstorming; branching.**

Minutes   These record what happen in a meeting, but in a rarefied way that makes them a prime example of **political writing**. Organizations will vary in their preference of **style** and **structure**, though most will encourage the use of the **passive voice**.

One of the hardest parts of writing minutes is defining how they can be seen as successful, or not. One of the certainties, however, is that at the next meeting someone will complain about the accuracy (not that they are inaccurate; the complaint is usually made for completely different reasons). This should be taken as part of the game, and not an indication of failure. A better indicator is whether the chair (or whoever is holding the meeting) is happy with them. In some organizations, particularly those with a full-time secretariat, writers of minutes may find themselves torn between the chair and their head of department.

For these reasons, use **action lists** wherever possible.

Misprints   Words on the printed page that have turned out wrong. These can give great pleasure, as in 'the vicar ran for a male' or 'We went to Pisa for a wee and half' (*see* **law of late literals; proof-reading**).

Mission   A few centuries ago this word (derived from the Latin verb 'to send') was used to describe a group of people dispatched overseas to conduct diplomatic negotiations. Later it was adapted to describe those sent overseas to spread a religious message. Over the past decade or so it has been adapted yet again, to describe the practice of writing down the purpose of an organization: 'Our mission at St Bede's is to treat people with hand injuries, preferably within four hours of arrival.'

Mission statements produce a strong reaction among medical folk, probably because many of them are written by **committees,** badly. For example: 'Our Mission in the Human Resources Division at St Bede's NHS Healthcare Trust is to foster and encourage the development of Individuals and Teams throughout the Organization in order to effectively satisfy the needs and priorities of those entrusted to their care, and to empower individuals and teams in a proactive, fulfilling and measurable manner.'

But strip away the pomposities and the platitudes, and there is a good idea in there. When you carry out a group activity, it is a good idea to sit down beforehand and work out what you are trying to do. A well-written mission statement (call it something else, if you wish) should clarify, not confuse. It should also improve the likelihood of everyone working together for the same end.

Monologophobia   A term first coined by Harold Evans, distinguished editor of the *London Sunday Times*. It is the fear of using the same word more than once within several lines of itself.

This fear is common. Some people, doubtless conditioned by a torrid time at school (*see* **post-spelling bee traumatic disorder**), feel that part of the challenge of writing is to find alternative words; otherwise others will think poorly of them. They may find these words, but often at the expense of making the text readable: 'The research indicated ... the investigations resulted in ... it was discovered in the studies' leaves the reader not quite sure whether we are talking about one piece of work, or several. Often the repetition of a word is a strong sign that the sentence could be improved. One first step would be to turn any passives into actives: 'The study showed three things.'

If you wish to conquer your monologophobia, don't give it a thought as you do the first few drafts. As you come towards the end of the rewriting phase, you may wish to keep an eye out for undue repetition; if you give your writing to someone else to read, they will almost certainly point out to you if repetition is getting in the way. If they say you are repeating words (and it is annoying them), then do something about it.

In fact repetition can be a useful device to add emphasis. 'Try, try, and try again' works much better than 'Keep trying.'

'More research is indicated'   One of the great clichés in contemporary science writing. Yet there are few signs of this banal sentiment disappearing. At least authors are starting to dress it up, moving from the relatively simple 'This study demonstrates the urgent need for further investigation ...' to the more ingenious 'Further analysis of the pharmacology will be required to further elucidate the exact role of this mechanism following this type of insult' or 'Further investigations are needed employing various transgenic mice to completely clarify this mechanism.'

For a more powerful conclusion, avoid concluding with the predictable wish that your researches be allowed to continue. Instead give the **message** – a simple sentence outlining the implication of what you have found (*see* **final sentences**).

Multi-authored books   These abound (*see* **books, editing of**; **books, writing chapters in**).

Myths   These abound when it comes to defining what makes 'good' writing. *See* **evidence-based writing**.

Names   The only thing more important than getting these (and the titles that accompany them) right is making sure you publish the right dosages.

Negatives   Prefer to say what is rather than what is not (*see* **positives**). Avoid strings of negatives – such as this one, found in an early-ish draft of this book: 'Don't automatically think that because you don't like what is written it will not have any good effects.' *See also* **double negatives**.

Negotiating changes   When we ask friends or colleagues to give us feedback on what we have written, we do not have to negotiate, because we do not have to follow their suggestions. When we submit our writing to co-authors and bosses, however, the situation is different. We have a formal relationship with these people. It is therefore not always possible to dismiss their proposed changes out of hand, even if we have reason to believe that these changes will ruin any chance our writing might have of putting our message across to the target audience (*see* **false feedback loop; proofreading**).

This is therefore a key part of the writing process, and should be approached with care. It will help enormously if you have already agreed with these people the overall message and the market (*see* **brief setting**). But they are still likely to propose changes: after all, it's seen as the function of a boss or co-author to make what they disarmingly, and often wrongly, call 'corrections'. My colleague Pete Moore has suggested a kind of triage, which divides comments from co-authors and bosses into three groups.

- *Changes that will help you to get your message across to your target audience.* Some comments will fall into this category. Incorporate the proposed changes, and thank your co-author graciously for the helpful contribution.
- *Changes that will have little effect on whether your message gets through to the target audience.* These are the most frequent comments, and they include adding unimportant matters of detail and substituting someone else's style for yours. Incorporate these changes also. As before, thank them profusely for their contribution – graciously, if you can.
- *Changes that will reduce your chances of getting your message through to the target audience.* These are the changes on which you must concentrate your diplomatic skills. Be rational, not emotional.

Provide evidence for your contention that the proposals could make the writing less effective. Ask for advice on dealing with this, though don't point out that the problem is of their making (*see* **evidence-based writing**).

Co-authors and bosses should not be commenting on minor matters, so as a long-term goal you should consider training them. Ideally, you should be in a position to hand them your work not for detailed textual criticism but to answer the simple question: 'Can you live with this?'.

If you are getting proposed changes from more than two people, you will find that some of the proposals are in direct conflict. In these cases you must assume a slightly different strategy. I would suggest two general principles: (1) try to negotiate away any suggestions that, in your view, are likely to turn off the target audience (*see above*), and (2) other things being equal, incorporate the suggestions from the most powerful adviser.

Newsletters   There was a time, as long ago as the early 1990s, when newsletters were all the rage. Anyone who was anyone had one, and at the first whiff of a communications problem, someone threw a newsletter at it. Part of the impetus came from the growing number of computer programmes that included templates so people with no formal training in editing could set up a newsletter. Inevitably newsletters began to fall into disrepute. A proposal to start up a newsletter was met by the comment, 'Not another!'. And everyone turned to setting up websites, which at least have the advantage that nobody can see them unless they actively search for them.

This is a pity because newsletters can be extremely useful. But they need to be well done: we are surrounded by high quality publications, and those that don't come up to those standards look tawdry. For those who still wish to persevere, here are some simple principles.

- *Do not set up a newsletter unless you really need one*. Don't just start because it seems (or someone else says it seems) a good idea. Define the need carefully – to improve morale, to sell more products, to encourage former students to leave lavish bequests (*see* **mission**)?
- *Appoint an editor, and give him or her space*. The editor should be responsible for all the content of the newsletter. He or she should be allowed to get on with this job, without interference. However, there should be a mechanism for getting rid of the editor if he or she oversteps the mark (*see* **editorial integrity**).

- *Set down annual schedules.* Many publications end after a few editions. This is usually caused by a failure to plan ahead. Work out how many editions you will have for the next year, and when you want them to appear. For each edition plan backwards with key dates, such as articles written, articles edited, articles laid out, completed pages to be printed (*see* **deadlines**).

- *Lay down a structure for the publication.* Work out which items will go where, not just for the first edition, but for subsequent editions as well. For example, put news stories on the first page, editorial and letters on the second page, a feature article on page three and some smaller items of interest and a mini-profile on the back page. Alter the running order with reluctance: readers like stability because it helps them find their way around. It also helps editors by enabling them to collect specifically for each section (*see* **commissioning**).

- *Keep the design simple.* Producing a newsletter should not be a way of showing off what your new computer can do. Design is a means to an end, and that end is to get people to (1) recognize the publication (hence the need for consistency) and (2) read items contained therein (hence the need for clarity and display). Choose a **layout** that you can use without too much trouble.

- *Write for the real readers.* This sounds obvious, but many newsletters end up being written for the 'wrong' people – the management team, for instance, rather than the average employee, or health professionals rather than patients (*see* **committees; false feedback loop**). Try to attract their attention with **intros** and **headlines**. Separate fact from comment (*see* **Pravda effect**).

- *Measure what you are doing.* Surveys generally have a poor response rate, with a bias towards the discontented. Consider performance measures instead: are more people phoning the help-line you have publicized, for instance, or are the GPs getting fewer trivial phone calls after hours? It's not always possible to have such definite measures, but if you are setting up a newsletter to achieve something (better morale, more sales, fewer nuisance telephone calls), you should be able to work out some way of recognizing when you get there. Other techniques could include observing how piles of the newsletter go down (and the contents of the waste paper baskets fill up!). If the newsletter is not working, have the courage to propose closure.

- *Trumpet your successes.* Keep reminding readers why they have made a good decision to read the newsletter. This could be some bare facts about how many people now receive it, **letters to the editor** (even negative ones show that the publication is read) – or a success story from a previous issue: 'Anne Smith lost her left shoe – but within minutes of this newsletter coming out she was reunited with it ...', etc. If you win a prize, don't be bashful – report it.

- *Identify the next editor.* Choose and groom a successor. A newsletter that outlives the first editor is a real success.

Newspapers   Like newsletters, though more widely read and with greater resources. It's worth studying them to find out why (*see* **medical newspapers; tabloids**).

News pyramid   *See* **inverted triangle.**

News story   The currency of newspapers, and an extremely effective way of putting across a message. The key to the technique is to define the message or 'story' in the first sentence (*see* **inverted triangle**). This can be a problem to those who have been trained in science writing because they are unused to giving such prominence to single messages (*see* **IMRAD structure**). But that's not sufficient reason to dismiss what can be a very effective way of putting information across.

Non-attributable information   The information given to a journalist on the basis that the source will not be revealed (*see also* **off the record**).

Not only ... but also   A **cliché**, though one of my favourites.

Nouns   Words that describe 'things', that would include people and ideas as well as material objects. Vivid writing contains many of them: bricks, pencils, daffodils, elephants, neurons, aunts, chopsticks, ouija boards ... the list is long and fascinating.

Noun salads   The practice of stringing together a dangerous number of nouns. This can be asking for trouble, as in: 'Hospital patient attendance officer returns audit.'

Novel   As in 'a novel treatment'. Somebody with a Latin education has written somewhere that this is the appropriate word to use for the advance described in scientific papers. Now it has become a **cliché**: everything is novel where I suspect 'new' would be perfectly acceptable – and more in line with current usage. Distinguish from 'the novel' – *see* **literature** and proceed with caution.

Obituaries   Obituaries are difficult to do well. You have a few hundred words to summarize a lifetime of achievements. You have to do this in a way that interests readers, most of whom until this moment will have lived in ignorance of the deceased. You will have to avoid giving offence to grieving relatives on the one hand, while avoiding conferring an instant sainthood on the other.

- *Make sure that you are fully briefed.* How many words and by when? If the publication provides written advice, make sure that you read it carefully. Look at other obituaries in that publication, noting particularly **first** and **final sentences, paragraphs**, and **style**. If you are unfamiliar with the publication, make sure that you know who the target **audience** will be.
- *Gather the facts.* Be inspired by what others have written in other publications (such as the daily newspapers), but don't rely on their accuracy. With the best will in the world (*see* **cliché**), mistakes get through, and the greatest insult is to carry them from obituary to obituary without checking. Speak to one or two colleagues or friends. Try to find an entry in a publication such as *Who's Who*; even better, see if there is a recent **CV**. Finally, speak to a close relative: don't worry that they might find it upsetting to talk. In my experience of writing obituaries for local newspapers, surviving relatives generally find it helpful to talk about their late loved one.

- *Work out the broad shape of the obituary.* Your research of the publication will have given you an idea of the number of paragraphs or sentences you will require. Write down three or four main areas you wish your obituary to cover: for instance, what were the formative influences? What were the main elements of the deceased's career? What were his or her other interests? And what will he or she be remembered for? Write in one go, without breaking off to look at the information you have collected and thinking of your target readers (not the family of the bereaved). Revise carefully what you have written, checking the facts you have cited, and making sure that you have not left out essential details (*see* **process of writing**).
- *Make sure you are using facts and anecdotes, not generalizations and bare qualifications.* Take out from your prose any unsupported value-laden words, like: 'gentle giant', 'well respected', 'much admired', etc. Make sure that you have put down facts and are telling stories. Use **nouns** and **verbs** to add colour: 'He was at Edinburgh for seven years where he became a familiar figure lounging around the Edwardian lecture halls in his pink waistcoat and green top hat.'
- *Check the facts with someone who will know.* In some ways the best person to do this will be a close relative. Here you must make it clear that you are asking them for opinion on matters of fact only. While you owe it to the family not to cause unnecessary distress, you also owe it to your readers to paint an honest picture.
- *Where appropriate, find a photograph.* The most likely source will be the family, though places of work could also help. Look for photographs taken by professionals, at an award-giving ceremony, perhaps, or even better at a less formal occasion and published in a local newspaper. Take care with your choice: it will be an enduring image. Make sure that the photograph is properly labelled: 'Joan Smith-Brown, pictured in the surf at a break during the Cornwall GP Trainers conference in 1983.'

One or two journals have experimented with the idea of self-written obituaries. These are generally accurate and unlikely to give much offence, but they tend towards extremes of undue flattery or unnecessary self-effacement. They have not become popular.

Off the record   An agreement between a journalist and a source that the information given cannot be published, ever. This poses all kinds of ethical dilemmas to a conscientious journalist:

what happens if he hears it from another person, for instance? If you want to give information, but not be linked to it (for valid reasons. not just cowardice), then speak on a non-attributable basis.

Be warned: there is a presumption among journalists that, as long as they have made it clear to you that they are a journalist, they will be free to report anything you tell them. It won't work to tell them a juicy story then add, 'By the way, that was all off the record.'

Ombudspeople

There is a fashion among publications to set up one of these. The danger in scientific publications is that they become yet another means of enabling disaffected (i.e. rejected) authors to take up inordinate amounts of an editor's time at the expense of the readers.

Omission, sins of

Many people find it extremely difficult to start writing because they fear that they are going to leave out something terribly important. Yet the things we agonize about leaving out are generally matters of detail, sometimes quite trivial. Concentrate on defining the message you want to put across – and then support that message in a plausible and readable manner. The material you then need to put in should select itself (*see* **process of writing**).

Openings

See **introductions; intros.**

Ordering information

Writing has a beginning and an end, so at some point in the writing process you must order the points you want to make in a linear form, by making a (preferably written) **plan**, noting down what you intend each **paragraph** to do. Before you get to this stage, however, I recommend a less rigid approach to organizing the material (*see* **branching**).

OPERA

Only Planning Ensures Real Achievement. One of those awful acronyms that comes from across the Atlantic. It is particularly galling, then, that the advice is rather good, and is particularly appropriate to writing (*see* **process of writing**).

Padding   If you are putting in extra words just for the sake of it, think again. Few people complain because they have too little to read (*see* **yellow marker test**).

Pain   Don't expect to write well without it (*see* **process of writing**).

Panic attacks   It is common to have these during the process of writing; after all we shall be judged on what we are about to write. There are two solutions: (1) walk away from the writing and do something completely different, or (2) get out paper and pen, or go to your word processor, and start writing anyway (*see* **writer's block**).

Paper   A medium whose time is up, possibly (*see* **electronic publishing**).

Paragraphs   The basic building blocks for most kinds of writing. A paragraph is a unit of thought and generally each should start with a key sentence, explaining why you are moving the argument forward (*see* **inverted triangle; yellow marker test**). If each point follows on logically from the previous point, then the paragraphs will also follow each other logically, and you should not find it necessary to insert artificial linking sentences at the end of each.

When planning a piece of writing, think in terms of paragraphs rather than words. Look at the market you are writing for, and get an idea of how many paragraphs the audience will be comfortable with. When drafting your plan, allow one piece of argument per paragraph.

If you are writing for a newspaper or magazine then your paragraphs will almost certainly be split up. This is done for visual reasons: long paragraphs and narrow columns are particularly reader-unfriendly. There is no point in complaining.

Passive   The passive voice pervades science writing, despite the pleas of many journal editors to avoid it (*see* **voice**).

Patient consent   Journals nowadays require formal written consent from patients who are being written about. Magazines and newspapers do not: their contributors are not normally bound by doctor–patient confidentiality. However, this does not mean that you should flout the rules of your profession. If in doubt, ask advice from a medical legal expert.

Patient information   If you visit any out-patient clinic you will see a vast amount of written patient information. In time some will be taken away and looked at; but some will remain gathering dust on the racks for months.

Yet, although some research seems to suggest that written information has limited value, the potential must be there. For those putting out the information, it gives the chance to consider what they really need to put across. For those of us receiving it, having it in written form gives us the chance to extract information at our own pace, without the tensions of a quick face-to-face interview.

Part of the problem seems to be that so much of patient information is produced by amateur communicators, breaking many of the guidelines long since accepted by professionals. If you wish to avoid falling into these traps, the following principles will help.

- *Work out exactly what you want to achieve.* Why are you producing your information? To make *you* feel better, or to produce some kind of tangible gain, such as patients feeling more in control of their condition? How can you measure whether you are achieving your goal? With fewer phone calls from worried patients, for instance, or evidence that they are taking their pills at the recommended rate (*see* **brief setting**)?
- *Check to see whether there is any existing information.* I constantly see people working hard on producing information that already exists in a better form already. This wastes time and money.
- *Suit the message to the audience.* This is not an examination, in which success depends on you putting out what you know. Nor is it a review article in a journal, giving an authoritative view of the latest research developments. Write for the patients and not for your colleagues (*see* **false feedback loop**).
- *Keep the language simple.* Avoid a posh overcoat and use the language of every-day life (*see* **pub test**). Avoid being **patronizing**, though that does not mean that you must avoid simple language.
- *Use illustrations.* Printing pictures, drawing diagrams and using other graphic devices will encourage more people to pick up your

information and read it. It will also help them to remember the information you put in it (*see* **layout**).

- *Control your costs.* The cost of printed information can vary enormously, and the key variable is knowledge of the techniques. Put another way, you can spend an awful lot of money and produce something that is unreadable, and spend next to nothing and produce something that does precisely what you intended.
- *Make use of your patients.* Even writers, designers and printers become ill. Don't be afraid to enlist their help. Usually they will be happy to advise out of goodwill; they may even find it therapeutic.
- *Test your information on the right people.* Ignore the views of your colleagues – their comments will almost certainly be criticisms of the content rather than judgements over whether you are getting the right messages across. Test any information on the target audiences – ask your patients to read it and then ask for their comments. You could gently probe them to see whether they have taken home the messages that you intended them to take home (*see* **payoff**).

Remember, this is not a test of your knowledge, but an attempt to put across some useful bits of information to people who are often frightened and confused, and delighted when they receive clear advice.

Patient's notes   *See* **case notes**.

Patronizing language   One of the problems of writing, particularly for patients, is that if you use long words you are criticized for not being concise – and if you use short ones you are criticized for being patronizing. This is an area where things may not be as simple as they seem.

The original meaning of 'patronizing' was to support (from the word 'patron'); somehow it has moved to a more derogatory meaning, which is to 'look down on in an obvious manner'. I find it difficult to believe that talking or writing simply, directly and honestly – writing 'use' instead of 'employ' and 'flu' instead of 'influenza' – can be interpreted by anyone as designed to make them feel inferior. The tabloids, for instance, use this kind of language – and are rewarded by millions of readers daily.

Where language becomes patronizing is not when the words are simple, but when certain phrases are introduced that define the reader as an outsider. Thus phrases such as, 'what we call', 'we doctors ', '[you] laymen '. In other words, there is an assumption that the reader will not understand.

The solution, I suspect, lies not in changing our style but in having a more robust attitude. If it is your target readers who are complaining, then you can easily make changes. But most of the accusations tend to come from those who have appointed themselves to be their spokespeople (*see* **false feedback loop**).

Payoff

Payoff   Too often we suffer vague feelings of anxiety about our writing. But writing can always be better. The question is: has it achieved what you want it to achieve? When it has, move on (*see* **effective writing**).

Pedants

Pedants   Those who get very upset when someone breaks the 'rules' of grammar that they were taught. Thank them, but then think **PIANO**.

Peer review

Peer review   The system of peer review started in the mid-17th century when scientists decided that, before they published an article, they should ask the opinion of others working in the same field. The assumption is that exposing work to the criticism of others will identify shortcomings and improve the quality of published material. It is a cornerstone of modern science publishing, with complicated structures developed to carry it out, and more recently a growing peer review research industry giving it added status.

Peer review systems vary, but generally, when a writer submits an original scientific paper, it will first be screened by one or two of the journal's editorial staff, who weed out the blatantly inappropriate or those that have disregarded the **Instructions to Authors**. Most papers go through to the second stage, which is assessment by others in the field who are known to the journal. Finally the editor, or someone to whom he has delegated this task, will decide, singly or with the help of a committee, which ones to keep. Normally there are more that have passed the quality controls than there is room to publish, so the final decision is generally taken on a subjective decision as to which one(s) are more likely to appeal to the readers (*see* **gut reaction**).

There have been three major international conferences over the past 10 years looking into peer review and medical journals. Much of this research has looked into the best ways of running the system, and into variables such as whether the authors should be told of the reviewers, or the reviewers be told of the authors, or whether young doctors from America make better reviewers than middle-aged professors from Europe (the evidence is that they do). Despite all the effort spent, there seems to be no 'best' way. Indeed many of the important questions – such as whether the system can be used to detect **scientific fraud**, or whether editors would make substantially different decisions without the system – remain unanswered.

All this, of course, is of marginal interest to most authors, who simply see the system as a major obstacle to publication. The system, for all its faults, is going to be with us for the foreseeable future, so the sensible approach is to learn how to manage it. Here are some principles.

- *Reviewers are advisers, not decision-makers.* The decision to publish rests with the editor and, although it will be helpful if you have pleased the reviewers, it is probably not a good idea to set out to do so. The reason for this is simple: you will not know who they will be. On the other hand, you do know who the editor will be – and by carefully studying the journal (*see* **evidence-based writing**), you will have a good idea of what he or she likes. So it is sensible to aim to please the editor – and hope that the reviewers don't mess things up on the way.

- *Don't get depressed when the reviewers come up with criticisms.* After all, that's what they have been asked to do. But it doesn't follow that their criticisms are useful, or even right, nor of course that they are always useless or wrong. Judge each comment on its merits and keep a sense of perspective. Try to distinguish between reviewers who throw in additional facts and tamper with the style on the one hand, and those who give useful **macro-editing** feedback on the other. If you feel that the final decision rests on a mistake made by the reviewers, consider appealing (*see* **dealing with rejection**).

- *The system is not fair.* Many writers spend hours complaining about the injustices of the system when they could be learning how to play the game. Editors and their staff may go to enormous lengths to ensure that they treat their contributors fairly. But, as long as journals are run as a business and there are more papers than space available, then the final choice will be made on commercial grounds.

- *Recommend reviewers when you can.* Some journals ask writers to recommend reviewers. You should certainly take advantage of such an offer. Tactically, you should include some of their work in the **references**.

- *Use the system to learn.* Flawed and misleading it may be, but it does mean that you get experienced people commenting on what you have written – and all for free. As long as you realize that these comments are almost, by definition, coming from a biased source, they can be extremely useful. In other kinds of publishing you will get nothing like this level of feedback (*see* **journal booklist**).

Perfection   The enemy of the published. James Thurber put it well: 'Don't get it right, get it written.'

PIANO   My very own acronym, and it provides a vital principle for effective writing: Put It Across Not Out. Actually it's quite hard to do.

Plagiarism   The practice of copying someone else's work and passing it off as your own. This is **scientific fraud**, and there is no excuse for it under any circumstances. Citing the good things others have said, however, is part of writing, and there should be no problem as long as you acknowledge clearly what you have done and have sought and received the appropriate permission (*see* **copyright**).

Plain English movement   This is the idea that everyone, especially those who draw up our laws and run our bureaucracies, should write in a way that everyone can understand. Groups have risen up in most of the English-speaking world to push for such reforms. In England the Plain English Campaign is one of them; for a fee it will put your text into plain English and award a crystal mark.

Yet somehow, despite the regular publicity, the notion hasn't really caught on, and with one or two honourable exceptions, much of the writing we get from large organizations is now as impenetrable as it was 30 years ago. Since most of us can communicate simply when we want to, it is not a matter of skill, but of culture and attitude. The question is not 'Why can't people write simply?' but 'Why won't their organization let them write simply? (*See* **political writing; putting on the posh overcoat.**)

Planning   *See* **time management.**

Plurals   *See* **Latin plurals.**

Political correctness   All around us are examples of how language is being deliberately changed to meet political agendas. 'Gay' no longer means happy and 'chairs' nowadays direct meetings rather than enable participants to sit down during them. Single word 'asthmatics' have now become the bulkier 'people with asthma'. *The Lancet*'s 'ombudsman' transmogrifies into an 'ombudsperson' when an article on the appointment appears in a US medical journal.

All this makes for easy targets. But, irrespective of whether we think some of the changes go too far, there is a valid reason for consciously trying to change the words we use. Language has a profound effect on how we view the world, and if we want social changes, then we must change the language being used.

For writers the implications are clear: using inappropriate words may cause people to reject your arguments and (worse still) stop reading what you have written. Clearly you should avoid them. But suppress any anxieties you might have about this during the actual writing stage. The time to take care of them is during the rewriting phase (*see* **micro-editing**). It doesn't matter if you appear to be an unreconstructed bigot at the first draft, so long as the final version doesn't give unintentional offence (though be careful how you dispose of the drafts).

If you are working in a particularly sensitive field, ask someone who knows about the political nuances to go through what you have written – and advise if you have inadvertently given offence. Writers should give offence from time to time, but it should always be premeditated, not accidental.

Political writing   This is the ability to take a simple statement and make it so hard to understand that the reader becomes confused. To achieve, this, ignore the normal rules. Take a simple statement. Add some peripheral uninteresting information and avoid using one word when several will start to confuse things beautifully. Use as many abbreviations as you can. Cast it all in the passive. Thus 'This pill may kill' becomes: 'It has been established in the scientific literature that there is a statistically significant relationship between a premature termination of life and the ingestion, by the generally accepted route and at doses agreed by the appropriate authorities, of this pharmaceutical product.'

The technique is extremely useful if you want to give the illusion that things are being done or that you are nicer than you really are. Some bureaucrats have raised it to an art form, but it is not **effective writing** as discussed generally in this book.

Politics of writing

When we write we literally put our thoughts in black and white, thus making us an excellent target for anyone who wants to criticize. Not surprisingly, writing often becomes a battleground, where those who have power give a hard time to those who might wish to wrest power from them in the future. Recognize these games for what they are: if someone changes your writing, it doesn't necessarily mean that you have got it wrong, or that they have done it better (*see* **negotiating changes**).

Polyfontophilia

The love of many typefaces. Modern word processing packages allow us to use a wide range of them nowadays, but this does not mean that you have to use all of them at the same time (*see* **typefaces**).

Pomposity

A disease of the over-comfortable, characterized by a tendency to use long words and needless phrases. Easy to cure (*see* **PIANO**).

Pompous initial capitals

There is great confusion over the use of capitals. Some people feel that an Initial Capital Letter conveys Dignity, and should therefore be used to describe People and Institutions whom we know and value. Thus we talk about Professors and University and Gynaecology and Resource Management Initiatives.

This is not an issue of **grammar,** but of **style**. Also, most research on writing shows clearly that capitals are hard to read and slow the reader down. They send a strong message that We are Important (though you, dear reader, are not). And when we start writing Consultants and Doctors but patients and nurses, then it risks becoming offensive – and therefore bad communication.

How do we resolve this? The most sensible principle is to use capitals for proper nouns (i.e. unique names) such as 'the *Daily Telegraph* Professor of Capital Letters at the Department of Pomposity in the University of Oxford' but thereafter, when the individual words become common nouns, use lower case – 'professor ... capital letters ... department ... university'. Committees sometimes get very tetchy about this; a good guideline is to put them in lower case if they can be interpreted as a common noun, for example 'a (and not the) finance and general purposes committee'.

Make an exception to this rule wherever there is likely to be major confusion. Thus use (upper case)'Trust' when talking about the group of people administering a hospital, in order to preserve (lower case) 'trust' for its traditional meaning of 'having faith in'.

Pompous words   These tend to be the longer words, and those coming from the Latin-Greek roots, such as 'commencement', 'participation', 'document', and 'residence'. Other things being equal (*see* **evidence-based writing**), prefer 'start', 'take part', 'report' and 'home' (*see also* **scientific words**).

Positives   Readers find it easier to cope with what is rather than what is not. Thus, 'He is calm and confident' rather than, 'He is no longer in a sense of confusion.' For **political writing**, however, ignore this principle: 'We admit that we are in deep trouble' can be replaced by 'We are not denying the negative impact of this failure to remedy our deficit situation.'

Post spelling bee traumatic disorder   The surprisingly common fear that, unless we can trot out long and obscure words – and spell them correctly – we will be judged as dunces. This has demotivated several otherwise good writers (*see* **macro-editing**).

Posters   A poster is simply a way of communicating information on a single sheet of paper, cardboard, etc. We are surrounded by them, which suggests that they are an excellent way of putting messages across (*see* **PIANO**). The medical and scientific community has adopted them as an important part of their intraprofessional communication. But in this context the posters are usually dull and badly presented, apparently favouring cut-down versions of the scientific paper (*see* **IMRAD**), rather than using the medium to its full potential. Content has edged out communication.

This makes it particularly important for those who wish to present a poster to work out in advance why they are doing it, and how they will judge their success (*see* **brief setting**). You may want to influence your supervisor, who will be at the conference, in which case you should look at his or her posters and follow that style. You may be wanting to impress the prestigious research unit up the road, in which case follow their style. On the other hand, you may wish to make an impact, in which case you should consider doing something fairly dramatic, such as limiting your poster to a photograph, one main sentence in bold type, and a few numbers.

Once you have decided what you want to achieve, you can start thinking about the mechanics. There are three main ways of producing a poster.

- *Solid panels*. Print out individual sheets of text and glue them onto large sheets of card. These can be difficult to carry.
- *Small cards*. Print out your text onto sheets of A4, enlarge them onto a clean photocopier to A3 and then get them encapsulated. This makes them tough and transportable – even in a normal-sized briefcase.
- *Print and roll*. Design your complete poster on a computer screen. When you have finished, send the file to a specialist printer who will print it out on a large sheet of paper.

In many institutions there are specialist departments who will construct these for you. They will normally have considerable experience of producing posters, and are worth listening to. However, you will be responsible for your poster, so keep the following principles in mind.

- *Don't overload*. Many people feel that being creative with a poster involves overloading it with text and different typographical devices. Look outside the academic world: use no more than two fonts. Avoid large sequences of words in capitals, or italics or bold.
- *Keep text to a minimum*. Posters are read (if at all) by people walking around. Trim your message to the bare essentials; this is not an examination but the communication of a message to someone whose feet are beginning to hurt.
- *Use illustrations if they add or attract, and not just because everyone says you should have one*. If you use illustrations make sure they are good, and that they are there for a purpose (e.g. to grab attention) and not just as 'wallpaper'.

- *Use the house style.* Many institutions have standard ways of displaying visual material. Both you and the institution will benefit from the continuity that a house style affords.

Finally, bear in mind that the poster is only part of the whole thing. You may be expected to make an oral presentation as well. Don't let the prospect of it spoil your trip (*see* **presentations**).

Pravda effect
This is the Russian word for 'truth'. During the communist era the newspaper of this name became a byword for biased stories favouring the controlling elite (*see* **propaganda**). All owners like to indulge their self-interest or vanity, as in publishing pictures of their own weddings or writing such blatant sentences as 'Our distinguished chairman drew on his enormous experience to give a most illuminating address.' But such a lack of self-restraint usually ends up making the publication a laughing stock.

Premature expostulation
Some people start writing as soon as they have an idea – and before they have done any thinking about that idea. This can be deeply unsatisfying (*see* **brief setting**).

Prepositions
These little linking words can cause huge amounts of aggravation. There doesn't seem to be any logic to when they are appropriate, so in most cases they have to be learnt. Here are some common problems.

- *Using the wrong prepositions.* Common mistakes include: 'bored of' (it should be 'with'), 'dissent to' (instead of 'dissent from') and 'centre around' (instead of 'centre on'). To some extent this is sloppiness, but there is also a question of usage. Sometimes these 'mistakes' actually represent changes in the language.
- *Different prepositions, different meanings.* There are several words, like 'differ', where the preposition can make a difference. (Use 'differ from' for comparisons, and 'differ with' a person.)
- *Prepositions at the end of sentences.* This was one of those rules to which English teachers were very attached (alternatively, and inoffensively, 'which they were attached to'). The latest Fowler (*see* **grammar booklist**) states clearly that this is a nonsense, and sometimes would be wrong. However, it also gives a warning not to leave the preposition 'stranded' from the verb (*see* **style**).

- *Prepositions that shouldn't be there.* There are some words, like comprise, which many people feel take a preposition, but don't,

Presentations

This is an essential skill for anyone wishing to impress (*see* **marketing**). Yet I have seen some dreadful presentations from senior doctors – too much information, badly presented with long lists of tiny type, or columns of endless figures written in purple ink and flashed up on the screen for about six seconds.

With a little time and care you should be able to produce a much better effect. Before writing the script, ask yourself some key questions.

- *What will the audience want to know?* How many people will there be? What kind of people will they be and how should you pitch the talk? What will they be interested in? What will they *not* be interested in?
- *How long will I have?* Allow roughly two minutes per slide, then leave a little time for questions. Identify in advance the slides you can leave out if you are running short of time. As a general principle, you will be surprised by how much you were unable to use.
- *Where will the presentation be made?* How far back will the audience be, and how will they be seated? What technical facilities, like amplification, will be available?
- *How will you judge your success?* A round of applause? Immediate promotion? The promise of a contract? Build in some measure by which you can judge your performance.

When it comes to writing:

- *Work out your key message.* Be absolutely clear what you want to put across (*see* **brief setting**) to the audience. And how you will judge your success.
- *Start and end with a bang.* Make a good impression from the start – and end with something memorable, though not so gimmicky that the audience forgets the main messages (*see* **first sentence**; **final sentence**). Show why it is worth listening to you.
- *Keep it short and simple.* Limit your ideas and limit your material. You will almost certainly run out of time.
- *Use graphics.* They are very powerful and audiences are now becoming used to seeing them. But make sure they are good graphics: nothing spoils a presentation so much as a visual cliché.
- *Be legible.* Limit the words on your slides and make sure that they are in large enough type to be seen from the back of the room. Edit

your figures drastically: people do not have time to look at columns of numbers.

When it comes to the actual presentation, bear in mind that all the careful preparation in the world is useless if the equipment fails.

Press releases   These are the tools by which non-journalists can submit news stories to newspapers and thereby place their own messages in the public domain, for no charge. They are potentially extremely powerful (*see* **tabloids**).

However, press releases can go horribly wrong. The tentative findings of a small sample study, for instance, will end up in the newspapers as a miracle cure – or a reminder to improve hygiene in the kitchen becomes an impending epidemic of killer bugs. Sometimes it is the fault of the journalist, who has been overzealous or misunderstood, but on other occasions it is clearly the fault of the writer.

Writing a press release is a completely different skill from writing a scientific paper. Here are some key principles.

- *Make sure you have something interesting to say.* Journalists receive dozens of press releases every day – far more than they have room to print. Most go straight into the bin. If you want a chance of being published, don't just ask 'Do we want to tell people about this?' but add the question 'Will anyone be interested?' If the answer is 'no', have the courage not to waste any more of anybody's time.

- *State the message clearly in your first paragraph.* Use a strong first sentence (*see* **inverted triangle**). Then make sure that the rest of the press release deals only with information relating to that message. Write five or six paragraphs of two to three short sentences each: if the journalist wants more then they will contact you. Include information only that is strictly relevant, otherwise you risk sending the journalist off on another story altogether.

- *Write the press release for the journalist.* Many press releases go down well within the organization that produces them, but clearly have nothing of interest to the publication's readers (*see* **false feedback loop**). The object of the exercise is not to please your boss or colleagues, but to get a story published.

- *Use an appropriate style.* Newspapers use a much different language from the one you are used to (*see* **readability tests**). If you do not translate, the journalist will. Phrases like 'using written communication techniques to modify the public health in a positive manner' will be turned into 'writing to improve public health'.

- *Use official notepaper.* Identify clearly that it is a press release from a reputable organization. Use double spacing. At the end of the text put a contact telephone number, and make sure that someone will be there when the phone rings. If you feel you must provide complicated background information, print this separately on a sheet headed 'Notes to Editor'.
- *Avoid propaganda.* Value laden words – 'We are pleased to announce the appointment of an excellent new director of public health who comes to us with a distinguished record of service' – will be destroyed one way or another. If you wish to include a value judgement, get someone to say it on the record (*see* **quote**). Make sure that it sounds like speech: nobody says things such as 'This is a significant addition to the organizational interface' (or if they do you should not spread it around).
- *Remain focused on what you are trying to do.* The purpose is to get some free publicity. If your story is published, then you have succeeded. Do not be put off by the inevitable criticism from those with other interests (*see* **false feedback loop**).

Process of writing

There are dozens of books telling aspiring writers what a piece of writing should look like after they have finished with it; few books tell them how to get there. Yet how we approach our writing has a fundamental effect on how it turns out. I believe there are five distinct phases.

- *Preparation: take time to define the task.* Writing often fails because we have no clear idea what we are doing, for whom and why. This is why it is helpful to spend some **rumination time** at the start working out the answers to these questions. You do not need to be facing a blank screen or empty piece of paper. You can combine your rumination with other things, like walking, or cycling or cooking. Resist the temptation to start writing too soon (*see* **premature expostulation**); instead, jot down the basics of your brief (*see* **brief setting**).
- *Organization: identify the information you could include.* Putting things down on paper is easy; the difficult bit is knowing which bits to put down and in which order. We therefore need a stage during which we formulate our argument and collect our information. This is better done before we start writing, and there are useful techniques (*see* **branching**) that can help us.
- *Planning: write down the key points that you wish to make.* Once you know what you could say to support your message, you need to

choose what you have room for – and how to order it. This means choosing an appropriate **structure** for your piece of writing, and then writing a simple **plan** outlining what each **paragraph** will deal with. Keep this very short: this is not a first draft but a route map that will help you on your way.

- *Writing: make the most of your creativity during the first draft.* Many people make too much of this part of the process, seeking to block off large periods of time, during which they sit and suffer and write painfully a few hundred words (*see* **writer's block**). But this is your chance to be creative not critical, and writers should let themselves go at this point, working in short periods of 15 minutes or so, encouraging creativity and suppressing the urge to stem the flow, to fiddle with the style or check the details of a difficult reference (*see* **free writing**).

- *Rewriting: invest time in improving what you have written.* This is a vital period, when we work on our first draft, making sure that it works on all major levels (*see* **macro-editing**) and that the details are also thoroughly checked (*see* **micro-editing**). The important thing to bear in mind is that this is an essential part of the process, and that time spent on this stage does not spell failure

One final point: we are all different, and can reach the same goal in different ways. It would be quite wrong to say that there is only one process, and that anyone who does it differently is doing it 'wrong'. What counts, after all, is the end product (*see* **effective writing**).

BOOKLIST: the process of writing

- *Writing on both sides of the brain*, by Henrietta Anne Klauser, New York: HarperCollins, 1987. A little gushing, but a stimulating look at the creative aspects of writing. She discusses some valuable techniques, like free writing.

- *The mindmap book*, by Tony Buzan, London: BBC Books, 1993. There are all kinds of non-linear creative thinking, and the technique of mindmapping, as pioneered by Tony Buzan, is one of the most developed. This book will explain how to do it.

- *Advice to writers*, by Jon Winokur, New York: Pantheon Books, 1999. A splendidly diverting and informative book. The author has chosen a wide range of comments, from one-liners to longer pieces, that are written by writers on writing. They will instruct, entertain and challenge.

Professors   They will usually have done quite a bit of writing. It does not follow that they are doing it in the most effective way (*see* **false feedback loop**).

Project management   Writing is not one task but many. Major pieces of work will need careful planning (*see* **time management**).

Proofreading   This is the task of reading a piece of writing that is about to be published, and identifying any errors that may have crept in during the writing and editing processes. The mistake that authors sometimes make is believing this is an opportunity for them to improve what they have written. It is too late for that, and any attempts to overturn previous technical editing will be distracting and dangerous – risking more serious mistakes. *See also* **negotiating changes**.

Find yourself a quiet corner so that you can give the proof your full attention. What you should be looking for are basic errors. Watch particularly for four types:

- *misspellings* of names of people or their titles;
- *numbers* that are inconsistent within the copy (i.e. literally do not add up), as in an early draft of this section, which urged readers to 'watch particularly for three types', while there were actually four!);
- *anything that could kill*, such as leaving out the 'not' in 'not indicated' or moving the decimal point on the recommended dose, and
- *nasty remarks* about other people that could land you in a court of law (*see* **defamation**).

Some say that you should read each proof twice, once for major errors and another for minor ones of spelling and punctuation. Others recommend reading backwards, so that you do not become distracted by the meaning. If possible, enlist the help of other readers: a fresh pair of eyes is far more likely to spot errors that you put there in the first place. Some people are better than others at proofreading: if you do find someone good at the task, cherish them.

Make your corrections clearly in the text. Most important of all, send the proof back in time for the **deadline**.

Propaganda   A derogatory term used to dismiss a piece of writing that we believe upholds a viewpoint with which we do not agree. (Writing that upholds viewpoints with which we do agree, we tend to consider fine writing.) All writing has some kind of bias, so we should not worry too much if others dismiss what we write as propaganda – provided that there are other outlets for them to express their points of view and that we have not done it too obviously (*see* **Pravda effect**).

Pub test   A useful and simple concept. When we speak we make use of a wide range of visual cues, such as eye contact and stifled yawns, to help us adjust to our audience and put our message across. When we write, we lose sight of the audience, and spend large amounts of time **putting on** (an unnecessary) **posh overcoat**. Whenever you come across a particularly impenetrable piece of prose that you have written, apply the pub test: how would you have explained this to your target reader, face to face? This invariably produces a sentence that is simpler and easier to understand.

The test is useful when helping others with their writing. Read the offending passage to them: 'The strategy has been designed to dovetail with the strategic planning processes of the main partners.' Cover it up, and ask what it means. You (and they) may well be astonished by the clarity of the reply: 'We need to consult with our partners.'

Publication date   The day on which a book, newspaper, magazine or journal will be published. Once this has been agreed, all kinds of other arrangements have to be made, such as reserving time on the printing press, and summoning extra staff to help with the distribution. Postponing these arrangements is tiresome and costly, which is why we need **deadlines**.

Publication planning   Many pharmaceutical organizations now spend time and money working out what papers they need to have published where and by when. Institutions and individuals would also benefit from this approach.

Publicity   It is probably an exaggeration to say it is *always* good. But it is usually less bad than many people think (*see* **false feedback loop**).

Pulse paradox   Doctors have been led to believe that the type of writing to which they should aspire is the type of writing they see in medical journals. But these articles are often badly written and hard to read, few take-home messages seem to get through (*see* CF Kellett *et al.* Poor recall performance of journal-browsing doctors, *Lancet* August 17, 1996), and it can take years for findings to be translated into action.

At the same time, doctors unite in their condemnation of medical newspapers, which they dismiss as 'comics' or 'funnies'. In fact the evidence of market research (and commercial success) shows that these publications, which are written in simpler English, are well read and acted upon. This leaves anyone writing for doctors having to choose: do they follow the style of the journal, and risk being ignored, or follow the style of the medical newspaper, and risk being undervalued? It's rarely an easy choice.

Punctuation   Marks that make our writing easier to read (*see* **colons; commas; dashes; exclamation marks; full stops; hyphens; quotation marks; semicolons**).

Puns   Using a word with two meanings and making people smile (or even laugh a little). The sentence or phrase should work with both meanings. Beware overuse: The write stuff (as a headline on articles about writing courses) has become a tedious cliché.

Putting on the posh overcoat   It is hard to escape the feeling that when we write we need to impress (*see* **English teachers**). So we can go to enormous lengths to make an understandable spoken sentence, 'Please turn off the light', into **gobbledegook**: 'It is recommended that the overhead illumination be forthwith terminated.'

Unfortunately this kind of writing usually ends up being incomprehensible, which leaves the clear implication that we need to put our messages out simply, without fuss (*see* **pub test**). There are clear exceptions – when writing for doctors who believe that writing is of value only when they have to struggle over its meaning. On these occasions you should write to impress (*see* **political writing**), but do not expect readers to act on what you have written (*see* **Pulse paradox**).

Quality   We all want our writing to have it, but what exactly is it (*see* **effective writing**)?

Questions   Starting with a question is a risky way of arousing interest. For all questions (even, 'Do you want to be rich and famous?'), some will immediately answer 'No', and read no further. As a general principle, only start with a question, or put one in the title or headline, if it is clearly the policy of your target publication to do so (*see* **evidence-based writing**).

Questions and answers   A dreary way to write up an interview. Interviewees favour them, because it gives them control; readers tend to switch off.

Quiet   You do not need to put aside large tracts of time in order to write. All you need is the odd 10–15 minutes and some sensible **deadlines**. So why not start now?

Quotes   Quotes are an important part of news stories. The function of the main part of the text is to relate independently verifiable facts: 'The new job will involve counting every paper clip in the hospital.' The function of the quote is to allow for comment or vividness: '"It is a vitally important job and we are so lucky to have Mr Smith, who has all the characteristics we need," said a spokesperson for the human resources department.'

Quotes can sometimes be controversial, with some people believing that journalists always make them up. Doubtless some do, but the majority will not. Unfortunately, many people don't remember what they have said, while others get cold feet, and change sensible statements like 'It seems hot' to 'There is evidence of an elevated temperature.'

If someone asks you for a quote, don't be flattered and accept immediately. Find out what they want you to talk about, who the audience will be, and what they really are trying to achieve. Consider whether you want to take part; if you don't do it, however, someone else will – perhaps not so well. If you go ahead, write down two or three key points you want to make. Be determined in putting them across: listen to how politicians manipulate (or even ignore) the questions in order to give the 'answers' they have prepared. Speak simply, and don't volunteer too much. When it is all over, be robust when others tell you that they wouldn't have done it that way (*see* **false feedback loop**).

If you are writing for a magazine or a newspaper then you may well want to use quotes from others. Make sure you have an accurate record, either as a written note or, more usually nowadays, on tape. Store these records for several years.

Quotation dropping   The practice of looking in a dictionary to find a quotation that can be plausibly put into the text in an attempt to show that the author is erudite. Adds little to the argument and is usually less a sign of erudition than that the author has access to a dictionary of quotations.

Quotation marks   Some publishers prefer double marks and others prefer single ones, so follow the style of your target publication (*see* **evidence-based writing**). Whichever one is favoured, use the other one for quotes within quotes: '"In a moment," he said, "I shall be boarding The African Queen".'

There is a tiresome point, much loved by **pedants**, of where precisely to place the **full stop** when using quotation marks. If this is the kind of thing that turns you on, refer to the **grammar booklist**. If not, put the full stop where you think it fits and let others sort it out.

Avoid putting single words that you think are slightly vulgar ('tummy', for instance) into quotation marks. If your audience doesn't know the word don't use it; if they do know it, use it without making excuses.

Quotations   *See* **copyright**.

Racism   *See* **political correctness.**

Readability scores   These grew out of attempts to measure how good we are at reading. They were first developed as 'reading ages' in the 1940s, but later lost their appeal – only to be saved by the emerging software industry which took several of these tests (such as the Gunning Fog and Flesch) and added them to word processing packages. They are entertaining and useful, though we shouldn't expect too much from them.

The Gunning Fog index, for instance, rests on the assumption that the longer the words and sentences the harder a piece will be to read. This seems plausible enough, though it leaves out a number of other variables, such as motivation and cultural background. Being numerical, it has a spurious air of scientific accuracy, and while a high score is associated with difficult writing, it does not necessarily predict it. Writing to keep the index number low will not in itself guarantee that something is readable.

That said, the tests can make an excellent market research tool that enables writers to test whether what they have written broadly speaking matches the tone that they are trying to achieve (*see* **evidence-based writing**). They can also show, when others try to change our work, whether they are taking it nearer to the style of their target audience, or moving it further away. Finally, readability scores encourage us to look at what we are writing in terms of how it will be understood – rather than whether we are meeting the rules of grammar and style – which must be a good thing.

Readers   These are what the writing business is all about. Without them we are wasting our time. So, to anyone reading this, thank you for bothering.

Readers' advocate   One of the most important tasks of the writer is to uphold the interests of the true target reader (*see* **false feedback loop**; **negotiating changes**).

Reading   An essential activity for those who want to write effectively.

Record keeping   It is prudent to assume that someone some day will challenge the facts that you have cited in your writing. Be prepared. Take good records of all you do – and keep them for several years. If you were challenged in a court of law, how would you fare?

Redundant words   *See* **flabby phrases**.

Refereeing   *See* **peer review; tautology**.

References   When writing for scientific publications (but not for magazines or newspapers), authors are required to give the source of any information or opinion that they cite, at the end of the text. These are the references, which are highly visible, make everything checkable and thereby, it is widely assumed, elevate the whole business of writing from anecdote and opinion into fact.

It takes up a lot of time, not only in reading, sorting and selecting, but also in negotiating which of each co-author's favourite studies should be included, and which others should be deleted. Authors can get bogged down with chasing and discussing references (*see* **writer's block**) sometimes at the expense of more important matters, such as whether the message is clear, or they are submitting to the right journal (*see* **brief setting**).

There is also a danger that the system as it now stands gives the illusion that science writing is more objective than it is. Often the references cannot be traced back and, when they are, the authors are clearly saying something completely different. In one famous study only about one reference in three was without error (George PM and Robbins K [1994]. Reference accuracy in the dermatologic literature. *J Am Acad Dermatol* **31**(i): 61–64). Bias creeps in because of the widespread use of the reference as an indicator of the worth of journals (*see* **citation index**). In order to keep their place in the league tables, wise editors make sure that articles from their own journals are quoted.

As for individual writers, they should consider the following principles.

- *Use the references to support what you have written*. Write first; add the references later. Do not write by collecting references into piles and then stringing them together into some kind of order (*see* **leaf shuffling**). By all means immerse yourself in the literature before you start to write, but during the **process of writing** make sure that references are kept out of sight. Add them during the **rewriting**.

- *Make sure you read every reference yourself.* This is an area where you do need to invest time. As the author you are responsible for ensuring that the references you cite are accurate, and this means reading them in the original as well as tracking them back to their first appearance. Be obsessive about this. It is unlikely that anyone important will check them, but there is an important matter of principle: how much value can we put on a system that prizes itself on its integrity when a major part is full of inaccuracies?

- *Follow the house style.* Read carefully what the **Instructions to Authors** says, and look at how references are handled by your target journal. Follow that style to the letter. You may be given the choice of using Vancouver or Harvard style. Ask your publishers to explain these if you are unsure. This will not only help you to create the right impression with the journal's staff, but it will also free them to spend time on more useful things, such as sorting out impenetrable sentences and double-checking the figures.

- *Use electronic reference managing systems.* It is now possible to buy software that will insert and arrange your references and put them into your target journal's style. This can save a large amount of time. However, don't use the ease of assembly afforded by these systems as an excuse for not reading the references.

- *Don't be shy about using references tactically.* Favour articles that have been published in your target journal. This will please the editors. It will also show that you are taking part in a continuing discussion that has been going on in its pages. If you are nominating reviewers, make sure that their work is cited.

- *Don't get obsessed with references.* If the editor or the reviewer disagrees with your choice, then you can remedy that easily. This is providing supporting information; it is not a public examination (*see* **false feedback loop**).

Rejection   This refers not to a general feeling of inadequacy (it's not really that kind of book), but to those specific and deeply memorable occasions when we submit a piece of writing, and it is sent back to us with a 'Thanks, but no thanks.'

The first thing to do is to grieve. Feel inadequate (though put a **deadline** on this). Go for a long walk. Otherwise do nothing that you might regret later. When you have calmed down, learn from what you have done. There is a good chance you will be able to get the work published elsewhere.

Don't blame others, or feel a failure. You have failed to 'sell' your product, so try to work out why the customer declined. If you are writing for magazines and newspapers, you will rarely have the luxury of detailed feedback, so examine the rejection letter carefully. The editor may have given you a clear reason, such as having a similar story already in the pipeline, or a judgement that the topic has run its course. But generally you will receive a bland and polite statement: 'I read your article with great interest, but I am, sadly, forced to the conclusion that publication isn't really a priority for us under present circumstances.'

If you are writing for academic publications, you will have the reviewer's reports to sift through. Make sure you work out the *real* reason for the rejection. Was it for technical inadequacies (in which case you should be able to take remedial action) or was it because the editor had other articles that he thought were more suitable for the readership (in which case you need to think of an alternative customer)?

Rejection requires one of three possible actions.

- *Throw the article away and try to forget the whole experience.* It is always tempting to do this, but consider how much work you have already done, and how much you are learning from the experience, painful though it may be. Persevere.

- *Appeal against the decision.* Another tempting option: all you have to do is write an eloquent letter showing the editor why the decision was wrong, and it will be immediately reversed. With magazines and newspapers this will get you nowhere: their editors will take the view that they don't advise you on surgery so they don't expect you to advise them on editing. With academic publications, however, there is the chance of appeal in certain circumstances. If the editor says that publication of your paper is not a priority then, as with the editors of magazines and newspapers, you must respect that decision (*see* **fairness**). However, if you believe that your article has been turned down because the reviewer has made an error and given bad advice, then you should consider an appeal. Do so politely, with facts not emotion. If the editor says that you are right but it's still not being published, respect the principle that the editor's decision is final.

- *Submit the article to another publication.* The preferred option. Under no circumstances should you just blank out the name of the first editor and send it off to another. Find a new **market** and research it (*see* **evidence-based writing**). Look at your **message**: is it right for that market or do you need to adjust it slightly? Go back to the start of the process (*see* **brief setting**). It will probably take less time than you imagine, and will be more effective than just tinkering with the rejected version.

When do you give up? Although most rejected articles are subsequently published somewhere, occasionally you will write the article that no one will ever accept. The logical time to give up is when editors and reviewers continue to make the same objection – insufficient numbers in the sample, for instance, or offensive to public taste – and you cannot (or will not) do anything about it. This is the time to hold a ceremonial burning – and get on with your life.

Most people receive rejection letters. While unpleasant at the time, they are good for the soul and better for the writing. And it does make that acceptance letter – when it comes – that much more worth while (*see* **acceptance**).

Reports   All professional people have to write reports. Generally these will review a situation (or problem), analyse it, and then put some recommendations. This is a specialized type of writing; once you master the technique, you have a powerful tool. Here are some tips.

- *Decide why you are writing the report.* Some reports, sadly, are written only because someone has been told to write them; these are pointless. Work out what you want to achieve. Are you reporting last year's activities, in which case what impression do you want to give? Are you writing to obtain an extra piece of equipment or new member of staff, or to change an existing policy? Are you writing to raise awareness of an issue, or to persuade people to take drastic action, like closing down a hospital? Whatever you decide, be clear in your mind how you will judge success (*see* **effective writing**).
- *Decide on the real audience.* Whom do you want to persuade that you have done a good job? Who will make the decision to give you more equipment or change policy? Who are the opinion leaders you need to reach? The more focused you are, the greater the chances of your report being successful (*see* **marketing**).
- *Sketch out the main sections you will use.* Examples might include introduction, background/history, current situation/problem, discussion, recommendations. Look at the reports that have worked before for your audience, and follow the style of the

successful ones. Approach each section as if it were a separate piece of writing (*see* **process of writing**).

- *Use the introduction to motivate the target reader.* Instead of writing, 'This report looks at a new cure for writer's block,' tell the reader what is in it for him or her. Thus: 'This report looks at a new cure for writer's block which, if introduced to this department, will ensure that our publication rate will treble' (*see* **first six words test**).
- *If necessary, write two reports.* Some documents run into trouble because they have to appeal, say, to an audience of professional colleagues who have one set of expectations (*see* **jargon**), while at the same time having to convince the non-professionals who will make the decisions. Fortunately there is a solution: write the report for your professional peers, and use the **executive summary** as your selling tool for the decision makers.

Research   All types of writing – not just science writing – will fail if the research is inadequate (*see* **bad writing**).

Research into writing   Even those steeped in the harshest traditions of evidence-based medicine can become remarkably cavalier when it comes to making decisions about their writing. But a wide range of evidence exists, both from psychological experiments into readability and from market research carried out privately for commercial publishers.

Here is a short selection of some of the main findings:

- *Long sentences.* Readers find it hard to unravel complex sentences. Making sure that the **verb** appears early will help.
- *Word choice.* Many readers' problems are caused by unfamiliar words, foreign words and negatives. Cultivate a simple style – and keep **positive**.
- *Signposting.* Readers find it helpful to have plenty of headings and subheadings. These tend to work better if there is a verb in them.
- *Typefaces.* The most important factor is that the type is large enough. For going across an A4 page, for instance, you should have a type size of 12 point. Don't mix too many type faces (*see* **polyfontophilia**) and avoid strings of capitals and long sections of italics.

BOOKLIST: research into writing

- *Designing public documents: a review of research*, by Elaine Kempson and Nick Moore, London: Policy Studies Institute,

1994. Useful advice for those designing forms and other documents, with details of many of the experiments on which this advice is based.

- *Designing instructional text*, by James Hartley (3rd edition), London: Kogan Page, 1994. This classic ranges over typography and layout, illustrations and tables, effective writing and evaluating design.

Resignation letters
These can be wonderfully liberating to do, especially when you are deeply unhappy. Say what you want to say, don't mince words, then put the letter away – at home. Do not store on computers at work.

Retractions
Be careful about these. They mean that you wish to take back an opinion you had earlier given. It begs the question: why did you say it in the first place? Distinguish from **corrections**.

Review articles
Traditionally they gave authors the chance to 'review' what was known on a topic, which involved assessing the information available, organizing it into a coherent structure, and drawing conclusions. This function is increasingly served by signed **editorials**. We also have **systematic reviews,** but these are written in the form of **scientific papers** and the term really refers to a research technique rather than a type of writing.

Generally authors will be invited to write review articles. If you are asked to do so, look carefully at other review articles that have already appeared in that journal (*see* **evidence-based writing**). Make sure you have in writing what the editor wants you to do – the precise topic, and in what form. You will also need to know such details as length, charts or tables, degree of original statistical analysis required, deadline for the article and other relevant conditions (such as will you get paid?). Ask for an example of the type of review article the editor has liked.

Look in particular at the structure: most review articles (though not systematic reviews) move away from the traditional **IMRAD** structure and follow the structure for **editorials** and **feature articles**. In general they start off with a first sentence that should attract attention, go on to set up the question they are to address, develop an argument that addresses it (one step per **paragraph**) and finally, at the end of the article, come to rest with the **message**.

Take time to review the material available before starting to write. Go through the normal stages (*see* **process of writing**). Be realistic about what you have been asked to do, which is to use your knowledge and skill to look at a topic, bring together the information you have found, and come to some kind of plausible conclusion. It is not the Gospel.

Reviews of books   *See* **book reviews**.

Rewards   Insufficiently used when it comes to writing. For major tasks (such as a **thesis** or a **scientific paper**) make sure that you celebrate as soon as you have finished. What happens later is, to some extent, beyond your control, though if all goes well you can have another celebration later (*see* **effective writing; payoff**).

Rewriting   This is a vital part of the **process of writing**. Don't rush into it: you will need to put some time between the first draft and this stage – preferably leaving it overnight, at least. When you come back to the draft you will need to look at it in a number of ways, though not necessarily all at once.

First, ask the **macro-editing** questions. These are the big issues, such as is the message still there, is it in the appropriate place and is it still right for the audience (*see* **setting the brief**)? Also ask if the structure works (try the **yellow marker test**) and whether the tone is appropriate? You will probably be surprised at how well you are doing so far.

Once you have carried out these tests, you can start looking at the **micro-editing** issues – **checking facts, accuracy, grammar** and **style**. It is important to get these right, but it is unhelpful to concentrate all your resources on them.

How many drafts should you do? There is no easy answer. Sometimes the number will depend on the importance of the writing – a **thesis** will usually receive more attention than a letter home. Sometimes it will depend on how well you have planned the writing. The big problem for most people, however, is knowing when to stop rewriting: this is where **deadlines** are invaluable. Printing out each edition as you revise will help to remind you that you are progressing a piece of writing and not just fiddling on a computer.

Some people feel that rewriting represent failure; on the contrary, it suggests that your writing is about to be successful (*see* **effective writing**).

Rubbish   There's a lot of it about (*see* **brief setting; crap**).

Rumination   The period at the start of the **process of writing** where you let the ideas go around in your head. You can do this while doing other things, such as riding a bicycle, lying in bed or taking a bus. Don't worry unduly if you don't seem to be making progress. But set a **deadline** because at some point you will need to put something down on paper (*see* **brief setting**).

Salami publication   The practice of undertaking one piece of research and then cutting slices off it for publishing in various journals. It is currently frowned upon by the editorial establishment. Editors take the view that the role of scientific publishing is to record and validate science, and therefore there is no reason to slice large studies into smaller bits. But, from the writer's point of view, the role of scientific publishing is to validate themselves and their careers, by enabling them to rack up points with each publication. So the more publications the better.

My advice to writers is to approach the matter from a different direction entirely. Once you have collected the data, define the **message** you want to give and match it to a journal (*see* **brief setting**). Then write your article, using the data needed to support the message. If you find, having written this article, that you have enough *unused* material that would support a *different* message suitable for *another* journal, then go ahead and write it.

Science writing   A term used by scientists to distinguish what they write from other types of writing which, by implication, are vastly inferior. There is no evidence for this belief (*see* **gravitas**).

Scientific fraud   A posh term for lies. There is no justification for them in any kind of writing. However, there has been a steady stream of cases over the last few decades, ranging from the slight (but nevertheless dishonest) massaging of figures to the lengthy discussion of patients that never existed.

Such cases tend to rock the scientific community, and there is now a widespread belief that the tradition of trusting other gentleman scientists is no longer enough. Editors are sensitive to the problem, and to the dangers of being required to spend more and more time policing science rather than communicating it. Academic institutions, therefore, are beginning to realize that they need to adopt explicit procedures if the integrity of researchers is to be accepted.

Writers should adopt the following principle: do not at any time put your name to a paper unless you are sure that everything in it is true – and that you could prove it if necessary in front of **lawyers**.

Scientific papers   Scientific papers contain original research, on a topic that is new and important. For many doctors and scientists they are the most important bits of writing that they do. They follow a specific formula (*see* **IMRAD structure**) and a particular style. They earn their authors valuable credits, which they use for climbing up the career ladder or amassing more funds for their department.

The question 'What makes a good paper?' is much harder to answer than 'What gets a paper published?' I therefore advise focusing on the latter (*see* **evidence-based writing**), because the task then becomes more manageable. Certainly it can be seen as any other transaction that requires researching a market, making a product and then selling it in that market. Meeting the following points should increase the chances of your article being accepted for publication.

- *Have one simple message to put across.* Often the starting point for a paper is the request to put a mass of data into some kind of order. Instead of immediately allocating bits of it to the four sections (e.g. details of the data collection into the Methods section), consider the work as a whole. **Ruminate**. Then set the **brief**, the first part of which involves formulating a one-sentence **message** for your work.

- *Decide in advance where you want the article to be published.* There seems to be a feeling that a paper that starts out suitable only for a minor specialist journal can somehow be improved by detailed criticism (*see* **Icarus fallacy**) so that finally it will be accepted by a major international journal. This is not so. You can and should decide, before setting out to write, which journal will be most suitable (*see* **marketing**). This will save time, increase your chances of getting accepted, and make the writing itself much easier (*see* **evidence-based writing**). Agree this with your co-authors before you start to write.

- *Collect information to support the message you have chosen.* The hard part of writing is not putting in information but deciding what to leave out. I therefore recommend some kind of brain storming (*see* **branching**) that will encourage you to select information that supports the message you have chosen. The advantage of this is that it also identifies what is not relevant.

- *Write each section in one go.* Many writers spend long and unhappy hours at a word processor, inching forward painfully. This produces demotivated authors and dreary, disconnected prose. Take your plan, find a quiet spot for 15 minutes or so, and start (*see* **free writing**), doing one section at a time. Never interrupt your flow – whether it be to go back and fiddle with the sentence you have just written, check a matter of detail with your records, or copy down the precise details of a key reference. You can do all this later.

- *Polish the draft and add the extra items.* Now you can start to work on the details, but be careful not to neglect **macro-editing**. Polish up the presentation of your figures and tables, and write the additional items you will need – the **title**, the **abstract**, the **references** and the **covering letter**. Follow the **Instructions to Authors**.

- *Handle your co-authors carefully – but firmly.* This is a dangerous time. If you have done your work well you will have a product that will meet the needs of your **target journal**. Yet many feel that they should now subject the draft to a barrage of detailed criticism, most of which will concern minor matters. It will be a great help at this stage if you have already agreed the market and message with your co-authors. Keep your nerve: your job is to keep the article on track for publication (*see* **negotiating changes**).

- *Send off the package.* Supply outstrips demand and your article may be rejected. If so, don't just throw it away (*see* **rejection**). If, on the other hand, your paper is accepted (as it should be if you have targeted it correctly) don't forget to celebrate.

Keep everything in perspective. The fact that you can write a scientific paper shows that you can write a scientific paper. It does not predict your performance as a doctor or your worth as a human being.

BOOKLIST: scientific papers

- *Winning the publications game* (2nd edition), by Tim Albert, Abingdon: Radcliffe Medical Press, 2000. Modesty forbids ... but this book takes the line that writing scientific papers is not as hard as many people make out. It goes through the process in 10 easy stages.
- *How to publish in biomedicine*, by Jane Fraser, Abingdon: Radcliffe Medical Press, 1997. Five hundred tips for success from an author who comes from the UK (as opposed to US) tradition of science writing.
- *Publishing your medical research paper*, by Daniel W Byrne, Baltimore: Williams and Wilkins, 1998. This book promises 'over 200 expert tips'. It is written from the US perspective and has some interesting data about what reviewers think.
- *Biomedical research*, by William F Whimster, London: Springer, 1996. A broad sweep through many aspects of planning, publishing and presenting research. Includes some useful chapters on the changes brought by electronic publishing.
- *How to write and publish a scientific paper* (3rd edition), by Robert A Day, Cambridge: Cambridge University Press, 1989. One of the few books on this topic that is genuinely funny.

Scientific words   Some words are truly scientific, in that they describe precise things or concepts, such as 'tyrosine', 'autosomal dominant transmission' or 'multivariate logistic regression'. Other words, such as 'approximately' (instead of 'about'), 'elevated' (instead of 'raised') and 'demonstrated' (instead of 'showed') are merely **pompous words**. Avoid them, even when writing scientific papers.

Semicolons   If you are having to look this up, don't use them (*see* **full stops**).

Sentences Keep them short, simple and active. Put the **verbs** in early. Keep out subsidiary clauses and phrases; otherwise you will end up with something like this: 'These results, on the effects of treatments and risk factors in determining trends in coronary heart attack rates and mortality, which include some early surprises, will create considerable discussion and controversy amongst the world's experts, although further analyses remain to be done.'

Or this: 'To ensure that evidence from systematic reviews informs clinical practice in district general hospitals, we believe that those professionals who lead clinical departments should appreciate evidence-based medicine and how to incorporate review evidence into effective implementation methods to influence their staff, such as wall posters or practice guidelines.' *See also* **final sentence; first sentence; topic sentence.**

Sexist language *See* **political correctness.**

Short articles Do not assume that they take less time than long articles. The reverse will usually be true.

Shuffling data around One of the main preoccupations of those writing scientific papers. There is a better way (*see* **setting the brief**).

Simplicity A virtue in writing.

Slander A defamation which is spoken (as opposed to **libel**, which is written).

Spacing after a full stop Many who trained as typists on mechanical typewriters were instructed to leave two spaces after the full stop. Word processors are more flexible when it comes to spacing, and now the convention is to have one space only.

Spelling   This gives rise to all kinds of difficulties, mainly because people love finding other people's spelling mistakes and using them to imply that they are uneducated, ignorant and no longer a rival for the next job (*see* **politics of writing**). One of the problems is that English spelling has few rules, and those that do exist have exceptions.

Computerized spelling checks do help, and there is no excuse for not switching them on. However, they tell us only that we have a properly spelt word, and do not tell us if we have a good word in the wrong place. (While revising early drafts of this book, for instance, I came across 'a strong of nouns', 'collecting the date', 'piss the buck' and 'subsequent grips from rivals').

One of the best ways of improving your spelling is to read clear English. I don't necessarily mean the classics: airport novels, newspapers and magazines are quite good enough for this purpose. You need to be familiar with the shape of words, because alarm bells will start to ring when you see an aberration. You then need a good dictionary, and the energy and self discipline to use it.

Meanwhile, here are 10 commonly misspelt words (UK version). Get them right and you are already doing better than others: *accommodation, corollary, diarrhoea, inoculate, occurred, ophthalmology, publicly, resuscitate, separate, unnecessary.*

Split infinitives   This is where the two parts of the 'infinitive' form of a verb are split by an adverb, as in (and now famously) 'to boldly go' rather than 'to go boldly'. This practice causes some people to get upset. All writers on style, however, seem to agree that this rule is based on Latin grammar and was misguided from the start. If you want to split an infinitive and it sounds right, most modern authorities say, then go ahead and split it. If anyone complains, pass them a reference book and challenge them to find support for their position.

Starting   *See* **getting started**.

Statisticians   Most scientific journals now take statistics very seriously, with professional statisticians advising them at the highest level. We need to take this into account when writing for journals and involve a statistician at an early stage. Establish before you start whether you will have enough numbers from which to draw any meaningful conclusions.

But keep a sense of proportion. Endless statistics can impede communications. Unfortunately much modern science writing has become a succession of statistics that only the statistician and his mate understand. Use statistics to support the message, not to drown it (*see* **leaf shuffling**).

Stereotyping In writing, and in life, a great evil. Listen, and then report accurately.

Stet Latin for 'let it stand'. A common proofreading mark which means – ignore the 'correction'.

Structure It is easy to get so caught up in the meaning of a piece of writing that we take for granted the way the writing has been constructed – in other words the structure. Variables are likely to include: how long will the piece of writing be (**length**)? How will it be organized (**paragraphs; sentences**)? Should the message be at the start, or buried at the end (**inverted triangle**)? Will it follow the scientific **IMRAD** structure? How will it be labelled (**headlines; titles**)?

The structure to use is the one that your target audience likes and knows (*see* **evidence-based writing**).

Structured abstract *See* **abstract**.

Strunk Co-author with EB White of an excellent book on style (*see* **style booklist**). His name was adopted by the staff of the late lamented magazine *World Medicine* to describe the process by which a piece of incomprehensible pomposity was elevated into crisp prose by the skilful editorial staff: 'That was most sensitively strunked'.

Style (1) Ask a group of people to describe a 'good writing style', and they will come up with a number of requirements, such as clear, elegant, flowing, concise, etc. They sound good but, alas, are vague and unmeasurable. They do not give us anything concrete with which to judge. Worse, they allow those who write badly to justify almost anything they have written: 'I think it's elegant! And it flows.'

Some writers also feel that style is a mark of personality – that writing is a chance for us to show what we are like and, in this competitive world, we have to show off our skills. If you are planning to write a book that will win a literary prize then that view might be sustainable, but this book is not about winning a place among English literature classics. It is about the craft of putting together words in such a way as to enable you to put messages across to a target audience. Over the past 100 years or so writers have generally agreed about how to make this kind of writing work. These include the following elements: logically developing **paragraphs,** short and simple **sentences,** active **voice, positive** statements and sensible **word choice.**

They are all good tips, but they do not tell the whole story. If you look at, say, a scientific paper in *The Lancet,* you will see all of the above 'rules' broken constantly. So what then is an effective style? I favour a relativistic approach: *a 'good' style is the way a writer constructs sentences and chooses words so as to increase the chances of getting the chosen message across to the chosen audience.* In other words, for simple **effective writing,** style is not writer-related but reader-related.

At least this gives us a yardstick with which to measure style. When it comes to those endless discussions with **co-authors** or **bosses,** it gives an easy solution: allow any changes that are likely to improve the chances of putting the message across to the target reader; resist those that will have the opposite effect (*see* **negotiating changes**).

BOOKLIST: style

- *The elements of style* (3rd edition), by Strunk and White, New York: Macmillan, 1979. The bible.
- *Medical writing: a prescription for clarity* (2nd edition), by Neville W Goodman and Martin B Edwards, Cambridge: Cambridge University Press, 1997. A splendid attack on the pomposity of medical writing with some excellent examples and some sensible advice.
- *Waterhouse on newspaper style*, by Keith Waterhouse, London: Penguin, 1989. Trenchant views on writing from a distinguished playwright and journalist.
- *The Picador book of sports writing*, edited by Nick Coleman and Nick Hornby, London and Basingstoke: Picador, 1996. Forget literature; look at how skilled writers describe the games we play. And ask why science writing is so different.

- *The plain English guide*, by Martin Cutts, Oxford: Oxford University Press, 1996. An excellent handbook on how to avoid gobbledegook from one of the original leaders of the Plain English campaign.
- *Put it in writing*, John Whale, London: Orion Books, 1999. A new paperback version of a book originally written for the *Sunday Times*. Essays range from 'Being understood at once' to 'Sparing the readers pain'.

Style (2)   The set of rules set by a publication to lay down policy in some of the many areas where there are genuine ambiguities (Mr or Mr. for example, or -ise or -ize?). The thinking behind this is that readers care little about which version you use, as long as there is consistency.

Style guides   All professional publications will have a style guide, ranging from one or two sides of paper up to (as with the *Economist*) a major book that may be published commercially. All organizations where members spend large amounts of time writing would benefit from a style guide of their own, or they should agree on a reference book that they will use instead. This will defuse those endless and time-wasting rows over matters as unimportant as the use of a capital letter or the exact positioning of a piece of punctuation (*see* **Instructions to Authors; negotiating over text**).

Subeditors   Although they can be mocked by the flashy prima donna reporters, subeditors play an important part in the business of bringing information out promptly in a reasonably clear and accurate state. Like **technical editors**, subeditors are generally experienced readers and writers who can turn turgid self-indulgent prose (*see* **crap**) into something approaching clarity and even interest, as well as spotting (most of) the worst and most dangerous errors (*see* **lawyers**). This gives substance to the view that some kind of rewriting – and preferably by an informed third party – should be an integral part of the **writing process** (*see* **rewriting**). *See also* **copy-editors**.

Success   Make sure you define how you will define it (*see* **payoff**). And when you get there, celebrate.

Summaries   *See* **executive summary**.

Systematic reviews   *See* **reviews**.

Tables   For scientific papers, these are inextricably bound up with the text. In essence, the tables should give the information gathered, while the text should provide a reader's guide to the main implications. Journals will differ in their precise requirements, and you must look at your target journal's **Instructions to Authors** before embarking on time-consuming work. Similarly, when writing for any other market, such as books or magazines, liaise with your editor to find out how data should be presented.

Tabloids   It is fashionable to be dismissive of tabloid newspapers, but writers ignore them at their peril. Millions of people spend huge amounts of money each day to buy them. They then read them – and go away with the messages that the authors intended. Few other pieces of writing are so consistently successful.

Admittedly, the messages in these papers leave a lot to be desired, catering to the prurient – and meaningless to those who do not regularly tune into popular TV culture. But they use some excellent techniques, and these can be applied to other, less controversial messages. They include the assumption that words are worth putting out only if they are read (*see* **effective writing**), the principle of starting with the most important message (*see* **inverted triangle**), and the practice of using all kinds of devices to attract passing trade (*see* **layout**).

Target audience   *See* **audience**.

Target publication   The journal, magazine or newspaper to which you intend to submit an article. Choose it before you start to write. *See* **evidence-based writing; Icarus fallacy**).

Tautology   Saying the same thing twice over, as in 'young child', 'past history', 'vision for the future' or 'priority for action'. Avoid (*see* **absolutes; flabby phrases**).

Technical editors   The unsung heroes and heroines of science publishing – who spend hours at their desks working on manuscripts that are full of internal inconsistencies and incomprehensible sentences and making them, well, less full of internal inconsistencies and less incomprehensible. They will spend roughly half a day on each paper: they will check for errors, put the copy into the style of the journal (which gets particularly tricky when it comes to dealing with the references), turn it into reasonable English and sort out uncertainties with the author.

The work is similar to the work of the **copy-editor**, who is generally employed by a book publisher. It is very different, however, from the work of the **editor**, whose principal task is to decide what goes into the publication. It also differs in some ways from that of the newspaper or magazine **subeditor**, who start from the premise that the writing needs to be marketed and polished as well as checked.

Good technical editors are worth their weight in gold and there is a clear message for medical writers: cherish them. The editor may make the decision over publishing, but the technical editor will be the person who will quietly and with little thanks bring it up to the required standard. Unfortunately the egos of many writers prevent them from seeing changes as anything other than a direct challenge to their authority and talents. Such people would do well to reflect that technical editors spend all of their days working on scientific manuscripts, and will know far more about them than they do. *See also* **author's editors**.

Tenses   Choose one time frame and stick to it. It is obviously wrong to say: 'We experimented on 3000 rats. Half of them die.' However, science writing has a convention that the past tense should be used for describing what you did and found ('The rats died when we gave them the poison') while the present tense should be used for a proven (or generally accepted) fact: 'Rats die when given the poison'). *See also* **verbs**.

Thank you   These two words are probably the most powerful tool for improving the quality of writing. They are, sadly, neglected (*see* **commissioning**).

That/which   The rule is to use 'that' when it is defining or restrictive ('The bed that is broken must be taken away' – take the bed away) and 'which' for the non-defining non-restrictive ('The bed, which is broken, must be taken away' – take the bed away and by the way it happens to be broken). That said, few people seem to know or care nowadays, so does it really matter? (My **copy-editor** thinks so, but then that's her job!)

Them   This has now become a singular asexual pronoun, as in: 'If someone claims that they are libelling them'. Purists hate it, but it looks as if it is here to stay (*see* **political correctness**).

Thesis writing   The bad news is that these are very long, very boring and very important. The good news is that the person who will be reading it is not only required to do so, but is generally required to look for the positive as much as possible.

That apart, theses are similar to all other types of writing (*see* **process of writing**). Work out exactly what the requirements are. These are sometimes made explicit in instructions to candidates or similar material, but more often candidates have to work them out for themselves. Look at papers that have succeeded and at those that have failed, and try to find out why. In some cases it will be the content (lack of information, poor argument), but look also for other variables, such as **length**, **structure** and **style**. Here is some advice.

- *Don't be intimidated.* One of the major obstacles to writing a thesis is the feeling that it will be used to judge you, personally. In fact what people write in their thesis shows how well they can write a thesis. The task is not to become an expert on your chosen topic, but to produce a long piece of writing that will achieve your goal.
- *Spend time thinking about what you want to say.* You will need a framework for dividing up the work. To help you do this, formulate, then test, the **message** that you think you should give. This will help you to avoid **leaf shuffling**. Then use **branching** to work from this central idea outwards, so that the large amount of information you are gathering begins to form a pattern.

- *Plan how you are going to spend your time*. **Time management** skills are crucial. Start planning at an early stage. Work out how and when you are going to find the time to research and write. The normal type of **deadline** ('I will/must finish this thesis within eight months') is horrifying. Break the task into smaller tasks – periods for background, for thinking and planning, for the first draft, for the second draft, and so on. Put these deadlines in your diary – and work to them. Make sure they are realistic and achievable.
- *Choose your language carefully*. This is not the time to use plain English. One of the purposes of writing a thesis is to show practising members of the profession or discipline into which you seek entry that you know the jargon (or technical language) that they use. Look for the current buzz words, and scatter them with abandon (*see* **style; putting on the posh overcoat**).

Thinking   A grossly underestimated and underused part of the writing process (*see* **analytical skills; branching**).

Throat clearing   *See* **coughing**.

Time management   Writing is not one task; it is several. Those who write most successfully (have 234 publications to their name or seven books all on the same subject) are not necessarily the better writers – but they are almost certainly the better managers of time. Here are some tips for managing your writing time more effectively.
- *Set your priorities*. As set out so often in this book, the first step is to work out what you want to do, by when and why. Writing is a time-consuming business, so be absolutely sure that you have time to do it. If you decide to go ahead, commit yourself – set yourself a **writing goal** and write it down. Wandering around promising yourself that you'll do it as soon as you have time is a guarantee that you never will.
- *Block off time*. We all live 24 hours a day, and fill each one of them up. When you decide to go ahead with a major writing project, you must also decide how to find the time. What will you stop doing – watching a TV show, for instance, or sleeping between 6 and 7 in the morning, or reading a newspaper as you travel into work?

- *Do little and often.* These blocks of time need not be very long. It is difficult to block off two or three hours, but why not 15 minutes a day? You will be surprised how much you can achieve. It will also stop you getting bored (and passing your boredom on to your writing). *See* **breaks.**
- *Plan ahead.* Work out when you want the writing to be finished. Then work out the tasks that need to be done on the way, thereby breaking the large task into smaller ones. Record your progress in your diary.
- *Create the right environment.* Remove distractions. This means writing on a clear **desk.**
- *Build in incentives and rewards.* If there are other people involved in a similar writing project, arrange to meet regularly as a **writers' support group. Reward** yourself when you have met your target. And then set a new one.

Timetables   *See* **deadlines.**

Titles (to articles)   What is a good title? This is the kind of question that those writing scientific papers get terribly steamed up about. The answer is simple: it's what the editor of the journal thinks is a good title. Look in journals and you will see all kinds of different styles: the *BMJ* for instance seems to like colons, as in, 'Left handedness and writing styles: a randomized double blind trial'. Others like verbs (**declarative titles**): 'Left-handed writers are more likely to construct long and boring sentences.'

The implication for authors is clear. Do not write your title until you have written your paper. Then treat it as a separate writing task: look at the 'market requirements', then meet them (*see* **evidence-based writing; headlines**).

Titles (for people)   People feel very strongly about the position they have worked themselves up to, and therefore become touchy about how we address them. When it comes to titles (Dr, Mr, Professor, Lord) there are two guiding principles: follow the style of your journal and offend those you write about as little as possible. The first principle should always take preference (*see* **style [2]**).

Topic sentences   What Americans call the first sentence in each paragraph. These sentences define what the paragraph is all about (*see* **yellow marker test**).

Training courses   There are many courses nowadays on the skills related to writing and (as a course provider) not surprisingly I am in favour. But they are not cheap, and if you want to go on one you should first do the following.

- *Work out exactly what you want the course to help you achieve.* What are the problems you want to solve or the benefits you are seeking? Do you have an article you want to publish? Are you having a bad time from your boss because you do not write well enough (whatever that might mean)? Don't just sign up because the advertisement looks good: do so only if it meets the development needs you have identified. Read carefully the objectives of the course to see if they will help you to meet those needs. Review the needs annually.
- *If in doubt, speak to the trainer before you sign up.* The key to running successful training courses is to have the right people on the right courses, so it is in everybody's interests to get this right. Again be clear what you want to achieve: state your goal and how it could be met. Assess the answer carefully.
- *Choose the type of training that you will feel comfortable with.* Courses vary from those that bring in eminent talking heads to talk to groups of 100 or more to smaller workshops with fewer than 10 people and one tutor. Find out what techniques they will be using, and choose the type you feel most comfortable with.
- *Make sure that you cannot achieve your development goals in any other way.* Courses are not the only way to learn. There are many alternatives, such as books, job swaps, finding coaches and mentors, keeping your own development logs. These will usually be cheaper.

Travel writing   Going on holiday, like being ill, is one of the more interesting things that happen in our lives. As a result, editors are inundated with articles on these topics. Unfortunately, their interest to the writer far outstrips that to the reader. The market is overcrowded and those travel writers that do get published are either staff reporters on a sponsored trip, or talented professionals who make it all look deceptively easy. If you insist on writing about your travels, consider the following:

- *Decide if you are writing it for publication.* Most travel articles are commissioned in advance. Occasionally some publication or travel board might run a competition, but usually the chances of getting published are small. So why not forget about publication and instead write for yourself and your family – for the satisfaction of organizing your thoughts and of creating a memoir for the future?
- *Decide if you are going to write about your trip before you go.* If you want your writing to be more than run-of-the-mill, you will need to observe carefully, ask questions, seek out the unusual and take careful notes. This needs to be done at the time, not on the plane on the way home.
- *Grab the reader.* Do not start at the beginning ('As the plane banked in over the sweltering desert, my thoughts immediately turned to the two challenging weeks that faced me.') Instead, pick out a defining moment – an incident or a place or a person that you can describe, thereby attracting the reader, as in: 'What's a didger-eee-doo?" giggled the wide-eyed fresh-faced girl from Denver, Colorado ...'
- *Write for the reader, not for yourself.* Travel writing isn't about you, it is about where you have been and what is worth telling about these places. The trick is converting what has interested you into something that is of interest to someone else. Describe the differences.
- *Use nouns and verbs.* Instead of talking about the 'wonderful hotel', 'superb food' and 'breathtaking view', be specific. Talk about smoke-dirty oak beams and sky-blue clay tiles, trout plucked from mountain pools and fried with almonds and butter, the smell of lavender on garlic, the constant scritching of the crickets, and the waiter with soup on his tie who spent more time combing his hair than passing the gravy.
- *Read good travel writers.* Buy some of the books from the greats, such as Jan Morris, Bruce Chatwin and Paul Theroux. But also look at some of the shorter features in the weekend supplements: these may be competent rather than brilliant, but they have been published.

Troublesome words   *See* **confusing pairs; homophones; spelling**.

Truth   It is unwise to expect your writing to describe universal truths. Writing is a perishable commodity, and writers should be satisfied when they have a plausible idea, supported by reasonable evidence, presented in good faith (*see* **scientific papers**).

Typefaces   A lot of people have strong views about which typeface to use, but the current consensus is that, provided you use a familiar type, the type of type will be less important than the size of type you use (*see* **monologophobia**). For most middle-aged people, 12 point is comfortable. *See also* **layout**.

Be consistent. Never reduce your typeface in order to fit in all the words; cut the words out instead. Never show off (*see* **poly-fontophilia**).

UK-US English   This can be a major problem, though it is an area where people may find it easier to adapt if one of the Englishes is not their first language. I have so far been unable to find a simple book that will guide readers through all the pitfalls, but here are some useful pointers.

- *Same words, different spellings.* There are several groups of differences, mainly concerning the US English preference for fewer vowels. Thus 'honour' and 'labour' become honor' and 'labor', and gynaecology' and 'haematology' become in US English 'gynecology' and 'hematology'.

   The endings –ise and –ize seem fairly interchangeable (though the US, the Oxford English Dictionary and the housestyle of the publishers of this book favour the -ize). The word 'program' now has universal acceptance, particularly when it applies to computers. This still leaves the odd pitfall, like 'grey' (UK) and 'gray' (US).

   Nowadays of course the problem is much less than it used to be, because your computer program (**stet**), if handled with sufficient knowledge and tact, will automatically point out when your spelling wanders over to the wrong side of the Atlantic. That is good news, except for paragraphs like the two previous ones which, if you are not careful, end up automatically 'corrected', with the word 'program' persistently being changed back to 'programme'.

- *Same meaning, different words*. There are several major differences, such as 'queue' and 'line', 'nappy' and 'diaper', 'cot' and 'crib', 'chemist' and 'druggist', 'tap' and 'faucet', 'pavement' and 'sidewalk', 'autumn' and 'fall'. Thanks to films and TV, we tend now to have little trouble with them. There are some more subtle changes, however: UK English has 'anaesthetics', US English has 'anesthesiology'; there is 'got' (UK) and 'gotten' (US), 'aluminium' and 'aluminum', 'zip' and 'zipper'. 'Mad' is insane in UK English but angry in US English; in US English 'pissed' is angry; on the UK side it is a vulgar word for drunk.

- *Same words, different meanings*. A dresser in the UK is where you put your china, in the US it is where you put your underwear. In UK English 'suspenders' are used to keep up stockings; in US English to keep up trousers. A classic confusion is when pilots say we will be flying 'momentarily': the US English speakers understand this to be 'in a moment', the UK English speakers to be 'for a moment, only'.

- *Differences in punctuation*. Misunderstandings can arise with nuances of punctuation, often because people don't always realize that there are these international differences. UK English uses commas in lists thus: 'apples, oranges and pears' whereas US usage has 'apples, oranges, and pears'. UK English will use the lower case after the colon, as in 'Colons: a difference in punctuation' (US – 'Colons: A difference in punctuation'). US usage also favours capitalizing the words in titles (as in 'Patient Released Prematurely from Hospital'). The spread of US programs on computers means that some of these practices are spreading, whether we like it or not, throughout the UK and the rest of the world.

- *Two countries, two different styles*: It is generally felt on the UK side that Americans prefer a more expansive style. To some extent this comes from some of the words ('apartment' rather than 'flat', 'elevator' rather than 'lift'). It also comes from a feeling that Americans are more verbose and less Anglo-Saxon. Who knows?

This should not give major problems to those writing for international journals. If you have worked out in advance where you are to publish your article (*see* **brief setting**), then this becomes one of a number of specifications that you can meet without too much trouble. Do not get obsessed by it: this is not a test of international cross-dressing. If you don't get it absolutely right, a well-trained **technical editor** should be able to make the necessary changes quite easily.

On top of this, find a friendly and literate American (which shouldn't be too difficult), and run through your copy with them. Beware the occasional pitfall – my American wife worried for weeks because I had proposed building a dresser in the kitchen.

Uncommon words   You may feel that sprinkling your writing with these sends a signal that you are learned and cultivated. This rarely works. If you use uncommon words sparingly (one per item of writing), people may be fooled into thinking that you are clever; if you use more they will consider you pompous and may well stop reading (*see* **post spelling bee traumatic disorder**).

Unpublishable articles   Unfortunately some people feel that working long enough on a piece of text will increase its chances of being published (*see* **Icarus fallacy**). This is not true, and we can usually identify articles that stand little chance of being published before we start writing them (*see* **brief setting**).

Unpublished articles   Too many people leave lying around in bottom drawers articles that could be published if only they could just summon up that extra burst of energy. But many authors suffer from **demotivation**. Take out the article, go back to the first stage of writing (**brief setting**), match it to another market, and have another go.

Upper case   *See* **pompous initial capitals**.

Up-to-date   We should commit to print the latest information we have to hand. Some people use this as an excuse for not parting with the final version. But we can do only so much. It is often better to go for the 'latest reasonable' rather than wait for the 'final and definitive'.

Vancouver group   Legend has it that the impetus for this group came from a group of editorial secretaries, fed up with having to retype manuscripts that were doing the rounds from journal to journal. Whatever the cause, the first group of editors met informally in Vancouver in 1978 and now, under the formal name of the International Committee of Medical Journal Editors, they meet every year.

One of their major activities is producing the *Uniform requirements for manuscripts submitted to biomedical journals*, now in its fifth edition. These set up common guidelines for submitting to journals – all of the 500 participating journals will consider all manuscripts that conform to this common style. The group has also issued a number of statements on layout of **references**, and on contentious matters, such as redundant or duplicate publication, definition of a peer-reviewed journal, editorial freedom and integrity, conflict of interest, and confidentiality.

They are useful statements, and copies of the guidelines, which include the statements, can usually be obtained via a participating journal. Their main value is that they show clearly how editors think on all kinds of matters, from the setting out of references to the function of each section of a scientific paper. But when preparing manuscripts, authors should start with their target journal's **Instructions to Authors,** some of which will refer you back to the Vancouver guidelines anyway.

FURTHER INFORMATION
Uniform Requirements for manuscripts submitted to biomedical journals, International Committee of Medical Journal Editors, available from ICMJE Secretarial Office, *Annals of Internal Medicine,* American College of Physicians, Independence Mall W, Sixth St at Race, Philadelphia. PA19106-1572.

Vanity publishing   A phrase used to dismiss those who pay to have their poems and novels published. It is not yet used to describe the growing practice of paying to have one's scientific paper published.

Verbs   These are the 'doing' words (the Dutch call them 'work words') that turn a phrase or succession of words into a sentence. Take 'geriatricians', 'monkey wrenches', 'back pain' and 'hospital beds'. In themselves they mean little, but add some verbs and the story begins. For instance: 'Geriatricians should hit the hospital beds with monkey wrenches to avoid back pain,' or 'The geriatricians were hit with a monkey wrench and are now lying in hospital beds suffering from back pain.'

Verbs give direction to a **sentence** and are vital for formulating workable **messages** at the start of the **writing process**. They can, on occasions, cause trouble, particularly when it comes to writing scientific papers (*see* **tenses**).

Avoid turning vigorous verbs ('to inspect', 'to determine') into less vigorous and more pompous nouns ('the inspection of', 'the determination of'). Also be careful about turning nouns into verbs: we can probably get away with: 'We stretchered them to the city where they were hospitalized.' But sentences such as: 'We have all been obsessing about what we could have done differently' can seem excessive. We can usually find a more familiar way of saying such things.

Very   Should be used occasionally, which doesn't mean that you can overuse other words like 'exceedingly' instead.

Vocabulary   Most of us have quite enough to put our messages across (*see* **word choice**).

Voice   This is one of the most controversial areas of writing, particularly when it comes to writing for a scientific audience. Verbs can be in one of two voices: the active or the passive. The active generally consists of a subject, a **verb** and an object, as in: 'The doctor studied the chart.' The passive is when the object of the action becomes the subject of the sentence, as in 'The chart was studied (by the doctor).' The disadvantages of the passive are that it is longer and less vigorous, and can be harder to understand, particularly when the sentences start to get longer.

Yet many people believe that the 'proper' way for a scientist to write is in the passive. Thus 'I saw the patient' becomes 'The patient was seen.' This gives an appearance of objectivity, but it has left out an important piece of information: who did it? (For the cynical this explains why the passive is so popular: it implies objectivity while at the same time protecting anyone who was actually involved.)

Nowadays most writers on writing urge authors to use the passive sparingly. Yet it persists in the pages of journals. Younger researchers often report that their **professors** have changed their vigorous sentences back into the passive, because 'that is the way science is written'. It all becomes very confusing, so here are some guidelines. Use the passive:

- *if most of the articles in your target publication still use it:* look at your target journal and see what they favour (*see* **evidence-based writing**); specialist journals will tend to use the passive, possibly because they have smaller staffs and therefore less time to make changes of style;
- *in abstracts:* there is a convention that **abstracts** are written in the passive; follow this style;
- *if you want to avoid responsibility:* 'It was decided to send the patient home' may have distinct advantages over 'I decided to send the patient home' if there later turns out to be a court battle (but it is cowardly);
- *if you are writing minutes:* the convention is to write, 'It was agreed that ...' rather than 'Smith, Jones and Brown agreed that ...'; after all, the whole point of most **minutes,** as opposed to **action lists,** is that they give protection when things go wrong;
- *in the first sentence of a piece of writing:* sometimes it is necessary to turn a first sentence around in order to put the more interesting part at the start, as in: 'A 15% pay increase for all doctors was recommended by the Review Body yesterday.'

Otherwise use the active voice, which is particularly useful in the following situations:

- *when you need to get a clear message across quickly:* 'I will intubate' rather than 'Intubation will be started';
- *when you are asking for a decision:* there is a growing trend for executive summaries to give decision-makers the information they need; write these in the active: 'We need another portable x-ray machine immediately';
- *when you are writing a covering letter to an editor:* the article itself may be in the passive (*see above*), but you should never use that voice for the covering letter; be active: 'We enclose our study, in which we established conclusively that ...';
- *when you are writing for a newspaper and a magazine:* check first, but these publications almost always prefer the active (*see* **evidence-based writing**).

Wasted paper   Contrary to what most people think, the real wasted paper is not those crumpled up sheets that get thrown into the waste paper basket. They are those bits of paper that should be in the waste paper basket, but have been sent out to readers instead.

White space   Writing is a visual medium and, whether we like it or not, the way our work looks on the printed page plays a major part in the way in which the reader will approach it. Hours of agonizing over the exact words to use can be swiftly undone by thoughtless layout. One of the important considerations is where the words do not appear. Use plenty of white space to frame the words. If you have more words than you have room for, cut the words rather than take away too much white space.

Word choice   Avoid any temptation to show off (*see* **false feedback loop**) and don't be obsessed by **monologophobia** (*see* **post spelling bee traumatic disorder**). Select the words that will enable you to put your **message** across most effectively to your target audience. Keep everything simple: don't use a long word if a short one will do. Use **nouns** and **verbs** rather than **adjectives** and **adverbs**. Avoid **tautology, flabby phrases, pompous words, gobbledegook** and **jargon**.

World Wide Web   We can now use our personal computers to send messages around the world immediately and at little cost. This represents a major revolution in the way we use the written word. Potentially we are all our own publishers, which poses huge questions for, among others, those running academic journals (*see* **electronic publishing**).

As for the impact on authors, the major change is that vast expanses of material for research have been opened up, which they can roam without leaving home. They may need to adapt their writing techniques to take account of the fact that we do not use the computer terminal in the way that we use a book. But the principles of working out what the market requires will still hold true (*see* **effective writing**).

Whatever happens, it will not go away. Log on and start using the World Wide Web. You may find a useful starting point in www.useit.com. Or try me on: www.timalbert.co.uk.

Worried well   In writing, as in health care, there are many people going around feeling that they have major problems when it comes to putting out their thoughts. This is rarely so. What they are exhibiting is the pain that comes with doing a difficult job well.

Write, how to   *See* **process of writing.**

Writer   Someone who is involved in the creative process of making sense of a mass of ideas and putting them onto a piece of paper in a way that has a good chance of being read. It calls for individual suffering, and attempts to do it in small groups rarely work. Do not confuse writing with **authorship,** which is a claim to part ownership of a **scientific article,** and usually involves arguing about what someone else has written rather than doing any writing yourself.

Writer's block   A commonly used phrase that refers to the suffering we endure when we should be writing – and aren't. It may take a variety of forms, such as sitting paralysed in front of a blank screen, or more subtle displacement activities such as cleaning out the attic or searching for the one piece of research that will put everything in perspective. Though the symptoms are often similar, the underlying causes are various, and I have identified the following types.

- *Type I early onset writer's block.* This generally starts when we are required to do a piece of writing but have no firm idea where to start. The paralysis may stem from the fatal combination of a woolly **brief** and the need to start writing straight away. More often, it comes simply because we haven't done enough thinking. Don't panic; do something else for a while, while your subconscious brain gets to work on the problem. Then turn to the sections on **getting started** and the **process of writing**.

- *Type II early onset writer's block.* We may have a clear idea of what we are writing, for whom, and even why. We may also have done hours of high-quality gathering of information. But now the problem is fear: there is so much information that we are reluctant to make decisions about how to use it in case we make a mistake and are damned forever. A technique such as **branching** will help you get the mess of information out of your head and onto a piece of paper. Once you have done this, you should be able to plan the piece and start writing.

- *Perfect first sentence syndrome.* We have blocked off two hours or so of protected time and have moved to the word processor, surrounded with every conceivable piece of relevant information. Then we freeze. We cannot start until we have found the perfect first sentence, so we sit there ... and sit there. There are two solutions. The glib one is to start with the second sentence; this can be effective. An even better solution is to make sure that we know how we want to begin before we reach this point (*see* **first sentence**). We should then be able to get going immediately.
- *Boredom.* We tend to block off too much time for our writing. If we do anything (well, almost anything) intensively for an hour or so we become bored. One solution is to take a rest: go and do something completely different and preferably physical, like weeding a flower bed or scrubbing a floor, for 10 minutes. Another is to make sure that we allocate only brief periods of time – up to 15–20 minutes – for our writing (*see* **free writing**).
- *Mid-stream writer's block.* This is when we are in the middle of even a short period of writing, and suddenly we grind to a halt and cannot continue. This is probably nature's way of telling us that we haven't prepared thoroughly, in which case the best thing is to stop, take a rest, and go back to the beginning to set another **brief**. Don't panic: once we know where we are going, it will take only a matter of minutes to knock off a new first draft.

Do not regard writing block as a sign of failure; it is a sign that we are taking trouble to produce something worth while (*see* **process of writing**).

Writers' support groups   Never underestimate the difficulty of sustained writing, nor the speed with which the intention to write can dissipate. This is particularly true of major projects, such as scientific papers, major reports, or theses. Here the prizes go to the persistent rather than to the clever or the knowledgeable.

This needs organization and discipline – and also support. So, whenever possible, groups of writers should join together to give support and encouragement. After all, if it works for slimming, it should do so for writing, which is much easier.

There should be about half a dozen members in the group, and they should meet regularly, perhaps every two or three months. Members of the group should be roughly at the same stage in terms of writing experience, otherwise it will become an opportunity for political manoeuvring and showing off. It is worth taking care over the kind of things you will allow members to talk about.

- *Define group and individual targets.* How many papers will the group plan to produce within a year? How many papers will each member plan to produce? Which journals will they target and who will the co-authors be (*see* **writing goals; brief setting**)?

- *Set deadlines and monitor progress.* Agree on the deadlines that you will have to meet if the targets are to be achieved. Use the meetings to record individual progress. This is a good way of maintaining motivation, and ensuring that deadlines do not slip.

- *Pool information and solve problems.* Difficulties will surely emerge, whether they be technical ones such as using a particular piece of software, or more delicate ones such as persuading the professor to return the paper you sent him three months ago. It is surprising how much expertise can be found in a group of six people. Sharing problems and solutions will encourage the group to keep moving towards its targets.

- *Celebrate success.* Every so often, and at least once a year, the group should celebrate its success. Some may wish to set a league table of celebrations, so that the greater the success the better the party!

A final caution: these meetings should be used as an opportunity to discuss whether the work in hand is being produced, and not to discuss the work itself. There is quite enough textual flagellation about. If you allow the group to start getting involved in this you will usually end up with the work of those who have met their targets being criticized by those who have not. It will institutionalize the **false feedback loop** and ensure that the group misses its targets.

Writing   This whole book is about writing but there are main sections such as **advice on writing; bad writing; books, writing of; books, writing of chapters in; concise writing; defensive writing; efficient writing; free writing; research into writing; science writing**.

Writing for different audience   Not a specialist technique but the skill that goes right to the heart of **effective writing**.

Writing goals   Writing, when done well, takes up a tremendous amount of time. Invest this time wisely. When you start on a major writing project, do so because you want it to achieve something and not because you rather feel you should.

This means spending time working out – and writing down – your writing goals. *Why* do you need to write: to advance your career, to tell people about the interesting things you are doing, to see your name in print, to make money? The answer(s) should give you some idea of what you need to do: if you want to advance your career, you need one or two original papers in major journals; if you want to tell people what you are doing then perhaps a feature article in *Pulse* or *Hospital Doctor* – or a newsletter for patients.

Now decide on – and also write down – your objectives: what you need to do to meet these goals. A much-loved mnemonic in this regard is SMART; we go one step further with SMARTER.

- *Specific.* How will you define what you want to achieve? The clearer and more detailed it is, the better.
- *Measurable.* How will you know you get there? What will be the criterion by which you will consider yourself to have succeeded?
- *Realistic.* Is it possible to achieve what you have set out to do?
- *Time specific.* When do you want to have achieved this?
- *Evaluated.* When and how will you review what you have done and see whether you are meeting the goals, and indeed whether the goals remain the same?
- *Revised.* Do you need to change your goals and objectives?

Objectives that are difficult to achieve are: 'Write two articles for journals' and 'Read some more about writing.' Applying the above principles produces manageable alternatives.

- 'Complete the article already in draft and send to the *European Journal of Left-Handed Surgery* within three months';
- 'Do a computer search to identify a book that talks about writing style and read it before the end of this month'.

For the price of committing yourself to paper, you can transform your dread of writing into well thought-out, rational, goal-related behaviour. Your writing should thus be converted from a millstone into a tool.

Xenophobia   A deep dislike of foreigners. And (because I can't think of any other suitable words beginning with 'x') this concept can be extended to the feeling that, if foreigners don't write in the way we are used to, then their thinking can't be very good either. This is a particularly British attitude. We should bear in mind that most of us can't write good English anyway, much less have any success in a second language, much less a third or fourth.

Yellow marker test   Over the years I have found this simple test an extremely useful tool for understanding the structure of a piece of writing. All you need is a yellow highlighter and several paragraphs of text. Take the highlighter and identify those sentences that you think are more important than the others. Identify full sentences only, so that you will be able to read them in order and keep the sense of what you have written, albeit in abbreviated form.

You have now identified the writing's structure. It will be divided into (1) 'bones', those sentences that take the action or argument forward and which will be highlighted in yellow, and (2) 'flesh', those sentences that elaborate or support your argument and will have been left unmarked.

- *Highlighting the first sentences of each paragraph.* If you have consistently highlighted the first sentences of each **paragraph**, your writing will probably be well structured and easy to follow. This makes sense: paragraphs are the building blocks of writing, so putting the important sentences up front will define each paragraph and ensure that the argument develops in an accessible way. If, on the other hand, your writing is not easy to follow, the yellow marker test will give some useful information on what could be going wrong.

- *Highlighting the end of paragraphs.* This reveals the tendency of well-trained scientists to apply the structure of scientific articles (*see* **IMRAD**) to individual paragraphs. They start with a gentle introduction and build up eventually to an interesting bit at the end. The question to ask is whether the paragraph, and the piece as a whole, would work better if it were turned around? Generally it would.

- *Highlighting sentences in the middle of paragraphs.* Here it would appear that a key point has been buried. Would the paragraph work better if it were promoted to the top?
- *One or more paragraphs with no highlighted sentences.* What are these paragraphs doing? You may be giving the reader plenty of information, but without a framework on which that information can be digested. There are two main remedies: (1) agree that the unmarked paragraphs are redundant, so cut them out, or (2) write a new key sentence for the start of each paragraph so that the reader can understand why the information is there.
- *Paragraphs where nearly every sentence is underlined.* This is another sign of overload: if all sentences are of the same weight, then you are in danger of writing a shopping list. Writing a key sentence could do the trick: if you have six important reasons why, for instance, Monday is really Tuesday, then bind them together with a new key sentence: 'There are six reasons why Monday is really Tuesday.'
- *A series of bullet points where some are highlighted and others not.* This reveals a contradiction. A bullet point list implies that all points are of equal importance, yet the yellow marker test has shown that they are not. The remedy is simple: rank in strict order of importance or consider two or more lists.

The yellow marker test is particularly valuable when preparing **balanced feedback** for a colleague: if you feel that a piece of writing is not working, it will usually tell you why. It is a better use of time than fiddling with someone else's style (*see* **macro-editing**).

Zzzzz   Sleep: a precious commodity. Once you have written what you have set out to write, you can hope to have a little more of it. Enjoy: tomorrow could be another writing day.